FIBER FUELED DIET

Restore Your Health With Fiber Fueled Approach, Boost
Immune System, And Optimize Microbiome. Obtain The Plant-
Based Gut Health Diet To Lose Weight And Maintain Your
Fitness With Everyday Meal Plan of Delicious Recipes.

GORDON BENNETT

Cover Designer: Samuel Allen
Photo Art Director: Federica Kesh
Editor: Gordon Bennett
ISBN: Print | eBook

Table of Contents

INTRODUCTION

A significant number of us get less fiber than we must have to keep up the ideal health. For those with weight loss objectives, eating an inadequate amount of fiber every day is unsatisfactory and might prevent us from accomplishing our optimal weight. Among its numerous advantages, fiber can help diminish the danger of creating dangerous ailments and diseases and effectively push us to lose weight.

Let's explore the benefits of fiber along with its types that are soluble and insoluble fiber. How fiber builds our immune system? Also, learn what fiber fueled diet is and how it helps in weight loss. In this book, we will follow the everyday fiber fueled meals and recipes. Obtain the habit of an amazing 7 days fiber diet meal plan for weight loss. And learn many more biological terms that are necessary to learn for healthcare. So, let's get started!

OVERVIEW

Introduction of Dietary Fiber

Dietary fiber is a complex starch that can't be processed. There are various kinds of fiber; however, it is usually separated into two general classifications: insoluble and soluble fiber. As the name recommends, water-soluble fiber breaks up in the water, while insoluble fiber doesn't. Since insoluble fiber goes through our body unbroken, assisting with cleaning our digestive systems, it is otherwise called roughage. Fiber is available in all plant nourishments.

For what reason do we need fiber?

Even though it can't be processed, fiber has a significant part in our everyday diet. Fiber is so significant because it does three significant things:

1. Helps in absorption

2. Helps battle infection

3. Aides in weight the executives

Fiber assists digestion

Insoluble fiber remains in judgment in our stomachs and assists with wiping out our digestive tracts. As it goes through our body, it assimilates water. Dissolvable fiber gets separated once it arrives at our huge entrail. Normal microscopic organisms grow and increase on this separated fiber.

In general, fiber will slow the processing pace, prompting slower digestion of food from our stomach. It helps keep us normal and maintain a strategic distance from clogging. It does this by expanding our stools' mass, and delicate quality by increasing water ingestion and bacterial development portrayed previously. This increased mass makes stools be moved rapidly through the stomach, and because the stools are milder, they are removed simpler than littler, harder ones. At last, by assisting with keeping processing results moving rapidly through the digestive tract, fiber restricts our body's presentation to possible poisons.

Fiber and disease avoidance

While examination into the medical advantages of fiber is as yet being embraced, it accepted that it assumes a significant part in forestalling or controlling some intense infections, for example,

- Intestinal Issues
- Inside Disease
- Colon Cancer

- Bosom Disease

- Prostate Disease

- Coronary Illness

- Hemorrhoids

- Gallstones

- Diabetes

- Corpulence

Moreover, most nourishments rich in fiber are likewise low in fat and great sources of different supplements, which can likewise help prevent or control these and different genuine ailments.

Fiber and weight reduction

Fiber has been known as the weight watchers fantasy. Examination shows that individuals who abstain from food high in fiber have lower body loads, lower muscle versus fat, and lower weight lists. A few specialists accept that the high rates of largeness in the western world are to some extent because our eating regimens are ordinarily low in fiber contrasted with different areas of the world, such as Africa and Asia, where diets are transcendently plant-based.

Fiber is imperative to those of us with weight reduction objectives since it takes more time to bite, causing us to feel fulfilled sooner, fills our stomach, causing us to feel full more, causes us eat less food and swallow fewer all-out calories doesn't include calories because the body can't ingest it is found in nutrients normally low in fat and calories interferes with the retention of fat is found in nutrients that are pressed with energy and minerals.

The normal fiber taking of grownups in nations like Australia and the United States is around a large portion of the suggested level. The terrifying measurement is being made lower still by the individuals who are following famous low-sugar slims down. For example, the Atkins and South Beach consume fewer calories because these weight control plans confine nourishments normally high in fiber and other complex starches expected to fuel our bodies.

How much fiber do we need?

The Recommend Daily Intake (RDI) for dietary fiber is roughly 30g every day. Generally, well-known, exceptionally prepared meals don't easily have huge amounts of fiber, and accordingly, a significant number of us are getting considerably less than we should. In any case, with most things, it is conceivable to get an overdose of something that is otherwise good, and fiber is no special case.

Eating an excess of fiber (more than 50g every day) can cause the bowels and bloat's looseness. It can interfere with the body's retention of fundamental nutrients and minerals.

Instructions to get more fiber into our day by day diet

1. Increasing the utilization of complex sugars is the ideal approach to build fiber consumption.

2. However, our body needs an ideal opportunity to acclimate to increases in fiber, and too huge an increase excessively fast can cause bloating, loose bowels, gas, and distress. Since fiber assimilates water, we likewise need to build the measure of water we drink while increasing our day by day fiber consumption.

3. If we have to include more fiber in our everyday diet, it is significant that we include it steadily over various weeks to keep away from these issues.

4. Here are a few different ways we would all be able to get more fiber in our weight control plans and a rundown of the absolute best fiber.

Approaches to increase day by day fiber include:

- Eat entire organic products as opposed to drinking organic product juices
- Supplant white rice, bread, and pasta with earthy colored rice and entire grain items
- Pick entire grain oats for breakfast
- Bite on crude vegetables
- Substitute vegetables for meat several times each week
- Analysis with global dishes that utilization entire grains and vegetables.
- Eat less prepared nutrients for new food sources
- Top hotcakes with warmed organic product
- Sprinkle high fiber oat on yogurt, smoothies, and organic product dishes
- Top pasta with steamed vegetables

- Continuously eat a side vegetable with supper
- Eat the skin of prepared potatoes
- When feasting out, request an additional side of vegetables
- Include veggies, dried beans or grain to soups
- Use beans in stews
- Include oranges, apples, pears, or mangos to servings of mixed greens
- Nibble on low fat, (softly salted or nonsalted) popcorn
- Utilize low-fat veggie plunges and dressing
- Never skip breakfast
- Munch on grain
- Settle on bundled/handled nourishments that have the most fiber

The best sources of fiber include:
- Vegetables
- Entire grains items, similar to oats and pieces of bread

- Organic products (Blackberries, dried dates, raspberries, and so forth)
- Vegetables (Brussels sprouts, corn, parsnips, peas, and so forth)
- Entire wheat pasta
- Earthy colored rice
- Coat potatoes
- Peas
- Beans
- Lentils
- Nuts and seeds

The ideal approach to getting fiber in our daily diet is by eating the greatest possible combination of fiber-rich nourishments. While bringing more fiber into the eating routine, it is a smart thought to begin gradually.

Rolling out each improvement in turn, such as trading white bread for wholemeal bread, for instance, is an extraordinary approach and guarantees that our body has the opportunity to become acclimated to the change. Moreover, making little, moderately immaterial changes to our eating regimen imply that we are considerably more liable to stay with them.

Food marks and Nutritional Food

Perusing food marks and looking into the fiber substance of the nourishments we eat on the Nutritional Food is probably the most effortless approach to distinguish whether different nourishments contain a little or a great amount of fiber.

In Australia and New Zealand, items that guarantee to be high in fiber or a superb source of fiber contained in any event 6 grams of fiber for each serve.

High fiber nourishments or those said to be decent sources of fiber ought to contain at any rate 3 grams of fiber for each service, while items that guarantee to give fiber or be a source of fiber must contain at any rate 1.5 grams of fiber per serve.

Fiber Supplements

When we can't get enough fiber through our eating routine, it might be suitable to consider taking a fiber supplement. However, recall that new nourishments are the favored source of fiber since they contain other gainful supplements. Getting enough fiber is imperative to the health of all, yet it is especially significant if we have weight loss objectives.

The current addition to the Nutrition and Health arrangement is a thorough, yet versatile, manual for utilizing dietary fiber to administer health and ailment.

Dietary Fiber in Disease and Health covers all dietary fiber sources with attention to preventing and overseeing interminable illnesses. Every section contains a cautious investigation with numerous figures and tables of the latest human dietary fiber that examines and remembers explicit proposals for the fiber types and admission levels needed to prevent and oversee constant ailment and improve health.

Furthermore, doctors, dietitians, medical caretakers, nutritionists, drug specialists, food industry researchers, scholarly scientists and instructors, naturopathic specialists, and other health experts will be attracted to the viable, prepared to utilize data and inclusion of subjects, for example, the fiber in gastrointestinal health and sickness, the fiber in malignant growth anticipation, the fiber in Diabetes Type 2, and the fiber in body weight and creation.

Dietary Fiber in Health and Disease will hold any importance with doctors and other medical care experts in a wide range of claims to fame, including general specialists, oncologists, endocrinologists, and different professionals hoping to execute dietary exhortation as a feature of the patient therapy plan.

If we believe that we have to increase the fiber in our eating routine, it is consistently a smart thought to counsel a nutritionist, dietitian, or another reasonably qualified health proficient for help and advice. This book will clarify what fiber is, why we need it, what infections it helps battle, how it assists with weight reduction, and how to get a greater amount of it into our every day consumes fewer calories.

CHAPTER 1

How Does Fiber Fueled Diet Help In Weight Loss?

Getting to a healthy weight and remaining healthy is a significant method to prevent coronary illness, diabetes, a few cancers, and different serious conditions. A large number of us know firsthand exactly how hard it is to reach and keep up that healthy weight. Also, there's no lack of ways to try to reach that point: You can check calories, carbs, or concentrations. You can scale back fat or sugar. You can attempt quite a few well-known weight control plans that hinder certain food nutrients, or highlight only one. Any of these methodologies may work for you. Or then again, they may not — in large part since they are confused.

An examination distributed in the present Annals of Internal Medicine recommends that something as basic as intending to eat 30 grams of fiber every day can assist you with getting more fit, bring down your circulatory tension, and improve your body's reaction to insulin similarly as viable as a more convoluted eating routine.

Analysts from the University of Massachusetts Medical School contrasted two eating regimens' viability and help from 240 volunteers. Half were approached to follow the American Heart Association's (AHA) diet for preventing coronary illness, in which you attempt to eat more natural products, vegetables, high fiber food, fish, and lean protein yet additionally cut back on salt, sugar, fat, and liquor. The other half was approached to follow a diet regimen wherein the main objective was to eat 30 grams or a greater amount of fiber every day. Neither one of the groups got counsel or proposals for work out.

The entirety of the volunteers had metabolic disorder — that is, every one of them had hypertension, high glucose, and elevated cholesterol, and were overweight. This group of medical problems enormously builds the danger of creating diabetes, coronary disease, and stroke.

The members in each gathering arrived at the midpoint of 19 grams of fiber daily. The two gatherings shed pounds, brought down their blood pressure, and improved their insulin reaction. Those following the AHA diet lost more weight (5.9 pounds) than those on the high fiber diet (4.6 pounds). However, the two gatherings had the option to keep up their weight reduction for a year.

The aftereffects of the examination don't demonstrate that a high fiber diet is fundamentally acceptable (or better) for health than the AHA diet or the profoundly stylish Mediterranean eating routine.

It lets us know that one straightforward approach can have any effect and that empowering solid practices might be more powerful than demoralizing unfortunate ones.

"Notwithstanding weight control, higher fiber diets can likewise assist with the prevention of type2 diabetes and cardiovascular sickness," says Dr. Blunt Hu, teacher of medicine at Harvard Medical School and educator of sustenance and the study of disease transmission at the Harvard School of Public Health. However, he advised, it's ideal for getting fiber from food, not from supplements.

Adding fiber to your eating routine can be simple and delightful. A high fiber oat or oats with berries on top is an extraordinary method to begin the day. For lunch, appreciate a serving of mixed greens sprinkled with chickpeas or kidney beans and a few nuts (almonds, peanuts, pecans, or walnuts).

Make a sautéed food for supper utilizing a combination of vegetables, and top with pumpkin or sunflower seeds.

Snacks offer another chance to get fiber. Entire organic products, nuts, seeds, or a berry smoothie with wheat or flaxseed are acceptable choices, as dried organic products (prunes, raisins), popcorn, and bean plunges matched with veggies or entire grain saltines.

Good Sources Of Fiber		
Food	Serving size	Fiber (grams)
CEREALS		
Fiber One	½ cup	14
AllBran	½ cup	10
Shredded Wheat	1 cup	6

Oatmeal	1 cup	4
GRAINS		
Barley	1 cup	9
Brown rice	1 cup	4
BAKED GOODS		
Wholewheat bread	1 slice	3
Bran muffin	1	2
VEGETABLES		
Spinach	1cup cooked	4
Broccoli	½ cup	3
Brussels sprouts	½ cup	2
Carrots	1 medium	2
Green beans	½ cup	2

LEGUMES		
Kidney beans	½ cup	6
Lima beans	½ cup	6
Baked beans	½ cup	5
FRUIT		
Pear	1 medium	6
Apple	1 medium	4
Banana	1 medium	3
DRIED FRUITS		
Prunes	6	12
Raisins	¼ cup	2
NUTS AND SEEDS		
Peanuts*	10	1
Popcorn*	1 cup	1

CHAPTER 2

What Is Fiber?

Fiber is likely the least exciting word in the field of wellness and nutrition. Wouldn't you agree? It helps us all to remember those pasty powders we see advertised on TV, and it seems like such an exhausting method to add sustenance to our plates. As a whole, we realize we need fiber; however, what on the planet does that resemble on an everyday plate, and what are the advantages of eating a high fiber diet?

The normal lady needs somewhere in the range of 30–35 grams per day of fiber every day, and men need somewhere in the range of 30–45 grams for ideal digestion, weight, and heart issues. The dietary necessities for fiber set by the public government have changed throughout the long term however have would in general range somewhere in the range of 20 and 35 grams for each day.

Regularly, fiber demand is normally best anyplace somewhere in the range of 30 and 35 grams at the very least.

What does fiber do, however, and for what reason is it that significant?

Fiber is one of the essential pieces of an ideal nutrition plan since it does substantially more than manage our stomach related issues. A high fiber diet can shield you from becoming ill, overweight, direct your glucose, and even assist you with dropping undesirable weights without cutting calories!

Dietary fiber is a plant-based supplement that is at times called roughage or mass. It is a sort of starch yet, not like different carbs, it can't be separated into absorbable sugar particles. In this way, the fiber goes through the intestine moderately. In any case, on its excursion, fiber does a ton of work. The expression "dietary fiber" alludes to the inedible pieces of plant-based nourishments.

In different contexts, "fiber" may allude to plant-based material, yet when discussing nourishment, the expressions "fiber" and "dietary fiber" are regularly compatible.

Fiber is imperative to assimilation and normality, weight the board, glucose guideline, cholesterol support. It has additionally been connected to life span and diminishing the danger of disease. The Institute of Medicine has set a suggested day by day sum (RDA) for fiber consumption. Men ages 50 and more youthful ought to consume 38 grams of fiber for each day, and men 51 and more established ought to consume 30 grams. Ladies ages 50 and more youthful should consume 25 grams every day, while their more seasoned partners ought to have 21 grams. Most Americans don't consume enough fiber, as per the establishment.

Advantages Of Fiber

Digestion

Dietary fiber helps in improving digestion by expanding stool mass and consistency. This is likely fiber's most popular advantage. Bulkier, milder stools are simpler to go than hard or watery ones, making life more pleasant, yet also keeps up colorectal health. A high fiber diet may help diminish the danger of hemorrhoids and diverticulitis (little, agonizing pouches on the colon).

Heart health

Fiber likewise helps lower cholesterol. The stomach related cycle requires bile acids, which are made somewhat with cholesterol. As the digestion improves, the liver pulls cholesterol from the blood to make more bile corrosive, consequently lessening the measure of LDL (awful) cholesterol.

Glucose guideline

A meta examination of studies concerning the connection among fiber and blood (glucose) levels distributed in The Journal of the American Board of Family Medicine found that expanded fiber admission can decrease blood glucose levels during the standard fasting blood glucose test (a trial of glucose levels after a short-term quick).

The article demonstrated that degrees of HbA1c likewise diminished with expanded fiber. HbA1c alludes to glycated hemoglobin, which happens when proteins in the blood blend in with glucose. It is related to the danger of diabetes complications. Soluble fiber is particularly useful in such a manner.

Conceivable malignancy anticipation

The exploration has been blended concerning the connection between fiber and colorectal malignancy prevention.

While the National Cancer Institute states that a high fiber diet doesn't decrease the danger to a clinically critical degree, a 2011 meta investigation from the British Journal of Medicine found a relationship between oat fiber and entire grain consumption and diminished danger of colorectal cancer.

A later study proposed that fiber may aim this advantage if an individual has the correct kind and measure of gut microorganisms. Fiber normally responds with microbes in the lower colon and can, in some cases, age into a compound called butyrate, which may make disease cells fall to pieces. A few people normally have more butyrate creating microscopic organisms than others, and a high fiber diet can help empower the microorganisms' development.

Life span

As indicated by certain researchers, fiber could assist individuals with living longer. A meta examination of pertinent investigations distributed in the American Journal of Epidemiology finished up, "high dietary fiber access may diminish the danger of complete mortality." One ongoing examination recommends that oat fiber, from nourishments like entire grain bread, oat, and pasta, is particularly compelling. Over 14 years, the individuals who ate the most grain fiber were 19 percent more reluctant to death than those who ate the least.

Food sensitivities and asthma

New examination proposes that fiber could assume a part in preventing food hypersensitivities, the presence of which has since quite a while ago puzzled researchers. Once more, this hypothesis comes down to the collaboration among fiber and microorganisms in the gut.

Researchers guess that individuals do not deliver the correct gut microbes to handle nourishments regularly connected with hypersensitivities, similar to peanuts and shellfish. Without the correct microbes, particles of these nutrients can enter the circulation system through the gut—fiber aids in producing a bacterium called Clostridia, which assists in keeping the gut secure.

Economical

Similar thinking clarifies why fiber may help individuals with asthma. Undesirable particles getting away from the gut and entering the circulatory system can cause an immune system reaction like asthmatic irritation. A 2013 study found that mice eating a high fiber diet were more reluctant to encounter asthmatic irritation than mice on a low or normal fiber diet.

High fiber diet

Fiber is found in entire grains, beans, products of the soil. It is regularly found in higher fixation in leafy foods skins.

The high fiber diet plan includes:

- Lentils, which have 16 grams of fiber for each cup, cooked.
- Grain drops, which have 7 g of fiber for each cup. Grain biscuits are likewise a decent decision
- Berries like blackberries and raspberries, with around 7 g for each cup
- Apples (4.4 g)
- Pears (5.5 g)
- Split peas are loaded with fiber with 16.3 grams per cup, cooked
- Dark beans, which have 15 grams for each cup, cooked
- Lima beans acquire 13.2 grams per cup, cooked

- Pearled grain, with 6 grams for each cup, cooked
- Popcorn's 3.5 grams per 3 cups make it a fiber full bite
- Artichokes: a medium artichoke has 10 grams of fiber
- Broccoli has 5 grams of fiber when bubbled
- Turnip greens have 5 grams of fiber when bubbled
- Green peas have right around 9 grams for every cup, cooked

Fiber supplements

People who are trying to get an adequate amount of fiber in their weight control plans regularly goto supplements. While the addition of the supplement is not comparable to fiber from the entire diet, fiber enrichment can be useful for individuals hoping to direct their solid discharges or experience the ill effects of blockage.

They additionally have similar cholesterol bringing down and glucose adjustment impacts — if you can get enough of them. The supplement doesn't carry close to as much fiber as a fiber-rich food like lentils or peas, so simply sprinkling powder on your yogurt won't get you the fiber you need.

Besides, fiber-rich nourishments are uncontrollably high in other imperative supplements, which you won't get if you add supplements to a non-healthy diet. Fiber supplements can interface with specific medications, similar to ibuprofen, carbamazepine, and warfarin. They can likewise cause bloating and gas.

To get all the advantages of fiber, numerous individuals receive a high fiber diet. While consolidating more fiber into your eating regimen, start gradually, including 5 g daily for about fourteen days, the University of Michigan suggests.

Whenever expended excessively quick or in overabundance, fiber can cause bloating, squeezes, and even bowels' looseness. Let your body become acclimated to having more fiber.

The University of Michigan additionally prompts adjusting noncharged beverages with stimulated ones. Since caffeine is a diuretic that causes loss of liquids, adding an abundance of caffeine to a high fiber diet can cause obstruction. Focus on two cups of non-energized liquids for each cup of charged ones. Include natural products (particularly berries) for each dinner. Start the day with grain oat or oats and berries, Add beans or vegetables to a noon plate of mixed greens or soup, or have a bean or lentil burger instead of one with meat. At supper, include high fiber vegetables like broccoli, corn, and turnip greens to meat sauces. Consolidate with entire wheat pasta or earthy colored rice.

Low fiber diet

Once in a while, clinical circumstances expect individuals to embrace a low fiber diet in any event for a period. Those going through chemotherapy, radiation, or medical procedures frequently need to give their intestine a rest, as per the University of Pittsburgh Medical Center. Individuals experiencing Crohn's infection, diverticulitis, incendiary entrail illness, and ulcerative colitis keep up a low fiber diet for a more extended time.

Individuals on a low fiber diet should keep away from a high fiber diet that makes the intestinal tract work more seriously, similar to vegetables, beans, whole grains, and numerous crude or singed vegetables organic products, as per the National Institutes of Health (NIH). Refined grains, many cooked vegetables, and ready melons, peaches, plums, bananas, and apricots are still alright.

CHAPTER 3

What Is A Fiber Fueled Diet?

The vast majority of us have to eat more fiber and have less included sugars in our eating routine. Eating a lot of fiber is related to a lower danger of coronary illness, stroke, type 2 diabetes, and gut disease. In July 2015, Government rules stated our dietary fiber admission should increase 30g per day, as a feature of an eating regimen. As most grownups are eating about 18g day, we have to discover methods of expanding our admission. Children younger than 16 years don't require much fiber in their eating regimen as more seasoned youngsters and grownups. However, they need more than they get as of now:

- 2 to long term olds: need about 15g of fiber daily
- 5 to long term olds: need about 20g
- 11 to long term olds: need about 25g

Kids and adolescents are just getting around 15g or less of fiber daily. Urging them to eat many products of the soil and a smooth diet (picking wholegrain adaptations and potatoes with the skins on where credible) can assist with guaranteeing they are eating enough fiber.

For what reason do we need fiber in our diet?

There is proof that a diet full of fiber (ordinarily alluded to as roughage) is related to a lower danger of coronary illness, stroke, type 2 diabetes, and colorectal malignancy. Picking diets with fiber additionally cause us to feel full, while an eating regimen rich in fiber can support processing and forestall blockage.

Tips for building your fiber admission

It's imperative to get fiber from a variety of sources, as eating a lot of one kind of food may not provide you with a sound adjusted eating routine.

To build your fiber-rich diet, you could:

- Pick a higher-fiber breakfast oat. For example, plain wholewheat bread rolls (like Weetabix) or plain destroyed entire grain (like Shredded wheat), or porridge as oats are likewise a decent source of fiber. Discover more about solid breakfast oats.

- Go for wholemeal or storage facility bread, higher fiber white bread, and pick wholegrains like wholewheat pasta, bulgur wheat, or earthy colored rice.

- Go for potatoes with their skins on, for example, a prepared potato or bubbled new potatoes. Discover more about bland nourishments and starches.

- Include beats like beans, lentils, or chickpeas to stews, curries, and plates of mixed greens.

- Incorporate many vegetables with dinners, either as a side dish or added to sauces, stews, or curries.

- Have some new or dried organic product or natural product canned in a common squeeze for dessert. Since the dried natural product is clingy, it can expand tooth rot's danger, so it's better on the off chance that it is just eaten as a component of a supper, instead of as a between dinner nibble.
- For snacks, attempt the new organic product, vegetable sticks, rye wafers, oatcakes, and unsalted nuts or seeds.

The fiber in everyday diet:

Fiber at breakfast

Two thick cuts of wholemeal toasted bread (6.5g of fiber) finished off with one cut banana (1.4g), and a little glass of natural product smoothie drink containing 1.5 grams will give you around 9.4 grams of it.

Fiber at lunch

A prepared coat potato contains 2.6 grams with a 200 grams bit of decreased sugar and diminished salt heated beans in pureed tomatoes 9.8 grams trailed by an apple containing 1.2grams will give you around 13.6 grams of fiber.

Fiber for supper

Blended tomato-based curry cooked with onion and flavors (3.3g) with wholegrain rice (2.8g) trailed by a lower fat natural product yogurt (0.4g) will give you around 6.5g of fiber. Remember that organic product yogurts can be high in included sugars at times, so check the name and attempt to pick lower-sugar variants.

Fiber as a snack

A little small bunch of nuts can have up to 3g of fiber. Ensure you pick unsalted nuts, for example, plain almonds, without included sugars.

All out: Around 32.5g of fiber

Fiber on food marks

The above model is just a representation, as the measure of fiber in any food can rely upon how it is made or arranged and on the amount of it you eat. Most pre-bundled nourishments have a nutrition name as an afterthought or back of the bundling, which frequently gives you a guide about how much dietary fiber the food contains.

CHAPTER 4

How A Fiber-rich Diet Is Beneficial?

Eat more fiber. You've likely heard it earlier. Yet, do you know why fiber is so useful for your health? Dietary fiber — discovered fundamentally in organic products, vegetables, whole grains, and vegetables — is presumably most popular for its capacity to prevent or lessen clogging. However, a diet containing fiber can give other medical advantages, such as assisting with keeping up a regular weight and bringing down your danger of diabetes, coronary illness, and a few sorts of diseases.

Choosing a delicious diet that gives fiber isn't troublesome. Discover how much dietary fiber you need, the nourishments that contain it, and how to add them to dinners and snacks.

Advantages Of A High fiber Diet

A high fiber diet standardizes solid discharges. Dietary fiber increases the weight and size of the stool. A massive stool is easier to pass, decreasing your opportunity of obstruction. If you have watery stools, fiber may help harden the stool since it assimilates water and adds mass to stool.

- Keeps up gut health. A high fiber diet may bring down your danger of creating hemorrhoids and little pockets in your colon (diverticular sickness). Studies have likewise discovered that a high fiber diet probably brings down the danger of colorectal malignant growth. Some fiber is matured in the colon.

- Reduces cholesterol levels. Soluble fiber present in oats, beans, flaxseed, and oat grain may assist lower blood cholesterol levels by bringing down low thickness lipoprotein, or "terrible," cholesterol levels. Studies additionally have demonstrated that high fiber nourishments may have other heart medical advantages, for example, decreasing pulse and irritation.

- Assists control with blood sugar levels. In individuals with diabetes, fiber — especially soluble fiber — can slow sugar ingestion and improve glucose levels. A sound eating regimen that incorporates insoluble fiber may likewise decrease the danger of creating type 2 diabetes.

- It helps in accomplishing adequate weight. High fiber nourishments will, in general, be more filling than low fiber food sources, so you're probably going to eat less and remain fulfilled longer. Also, high fiber nourishments will generally take more time to eat and be less "vitality thick," which implies they have fewer calories for a similar food volume.

- It encourages you to live more. Studies recommend that expanding your dietary fiber demand — particularly grain fiber — is related to a diminished danger of death from cardiovascular disease and all cancers.

Advantages of a low fiber diet

Your body is the main "power" you can trust unequivocally. It allows you to feel and assess the upsides of a low fiber diet "by your gut." If that is insufficient for you, or if it appears to be excessively emotional, consider contrasting your past and current blood tests. You ought to watch a drop in your fatty substances and HbA1c (the average measure of glucose in the course of the last six to about two months), and in all likelihood, a rise in your HDL ("great") cholesterol. If you need to research things significantly further, request that your PCP audit you over a wide period of metabolic (kidney and diabetes-related) and hepatic (liver-related) test results, and you should see them normalizing too.

Simply remember that it takes years, maybe decades, to create diet-related health issues. Henceforth, it is unusual to anticipate that any eating regimen—low fiber or not—can mystically fix the entirety of the harm in a day, seven days, or even a year. In any case, taking everything into account, showing signs of improvement, even gradually, is a much better choice than wasting time.

So what's so mystical about a low fiber diet? Two things: (1) it makes the stomach related cycle fast and productive, and (2) it's normally low in sugars. Here's a concise summation of its most significant preferences. To start with, regarding your absorption. The benefits of a low fiber diet don't stop with simply done gorging. Here's a short recap of its other certain advantages:

Oral health. A low fiber diet improves dental health since it reduces bacterial aging inside the oral cavity. The side effects of maturation are the main source of dental caries (cavities), gum disease, perio-dontal infection, and tooth misfortune.

Throat. A low fiber diet prevents acid reflux. Thus, this eliminates the reasons for fiery esophageal disease (esopha-gitis), which may bring about the improvement of dysphagia (challenges gulping), Barrett's illness (irreversible difference in the esophageal epithelium), and malignant growth.

Gastric assimilation. Suppers without fiber and starches promote quick and complete stomach assimilation. The enhancements are especially clear in individuals beyond 50 years old (the gathering frequently influenced by acid reflux, GERD, gastritis, and peptic ul-cers).

Duodenum. A low fiber diet prevents duodenitis and duodenal ulcers. The all-inclusive contact of the duodenal epithelium with fi-ber absorbed hydrochloric corrosive and gastric catalysts is an essential driver of these provocative conditions.

Pancreas. A low fiber diet shields the pancreatic tubes from obstruction and resulting pancreatitis. Intense pancreatitis is the main source of type I diabetes indications in youngsters, whose little organs can get stopped up by fiber without any problem.

Gallbladder. A low fiber diet prevents cholecystitis, which is the hindrance of the biliary ducts, through which the gallbladder and liver release bile into the duodenum. Once more, fiber is the main external substance fit for causing the essential obstruc-tion (the optional block originates from gallstones and bile salts). Intense cholecystitis is the main source of gallbladder dis-ease brought about by gallstones, gallbladder inflammation, or both. Every year over a large portion of a million Americans goes through a cholecystec-tomy (gallbladder evacuation medical procedure). As you would anticipate, obe-sity and diabetes—the two conditions achieved by a high-carb/high fiber diet—are the cholecystitis' main sources. Also, truly, ladies are twice as likely as men to have gallstones. No sur-prise there: ladies eat more fiber than men since twice the same number of ladies are likewise influenced by clogging.

Intestinal block. Intestinal obstruction isn't possible with nutrients that digest totally. The small digestive organs should move fluid chyme just, not huge chunks of undigested fiber. Intestinal hindrances on a low fiber diet are as likely as a rain-bow during a storm.

Hernia. A low fiber diet prevents herniation of the stomach divider by the small digestive tract or its bulge inside the scrotum. These two conditions will probably happen when the digestion tracts expand past the stomach cavity limit to hold them. There is just a single food part fit for causing this sort of extension: toxic fiber.

Enteritis. Low fiber diet shields the intestinal epithelium from aggravation brought about by mechanical contact, from synthetic irrita-tion, brought about by gastric juices and catalysts (consumed by fiber while in the stomach), and from obstruc-tions brought about by chunks of fiber.

Lack of healthy sustenance. Enteritis, regardless of whether brought about by the mechanical properties of insoluble fiber, substance properties of soluble fiber, or allergenicity of plant proteins, hinders the absorption of nutrients, including basic, health-supporting amino acids, greasy ac-ids, nutrients, minerals, and microelements. This causes a wide scope of degenerative sicknesses, running from poisonous iron deficiency to kwashiorkor, osteomalacia to birth imperfections, and everything in the middle. A low fiber diet, particularly one liberated from wheat (a source of gluten), is basic for the best possible absorption of nutri-ents.

Swelling and flatus. The maturation of fiber inside the huge in-testine produces bountiful gases, which cause torment and bloating. A without fiber diet kills intestinal bloating and the source of the agony (from pressure). Flatus is especially troublesome regarding social associations for all individuals, and it's inside and out difficult for most. A low fiber diet lessens the presence of gases to the scarcely distinguishable.

An infected appendix. A low fiber diet is critical to preventing a ruptured appendix. The gathering of fiber inside the cecum hinders the appendix and causes its irritation. There is nothing that can cause a supplement check because, under typical circum-stances, the cecum's substance is liquid. Kids are particularly weak because their cecum is small, rigid, and inclined to ob-struction.

Loose bowels. A low fiber diet prevents loose bowels. No matter what, a wide range of dissolvable fiber is a looseness of the bowels causing operators. Therefore fiber is generally utilized in therapeutic and homemade diuretics. Intestinal irritation brought about by insoluble fiber obstructs the ingestion of liquids and causes loose bowels. Join the two aggravations, include (as generally suggested) considerably more fiber to treat looseness of the bowels, and you're guaranteed of the stool getting perpetual or transforming into ulcerative colitis or Crohn's sickness.

Obstruction. A low fiber diet wipes out obstruction brought about by huge stools. If you don't need your kids to encounter clogging, wipe out fiber-rich diet from their eating regimens. Unfortunately, a low fiber diet alone isn't adequate to treat obstruction after huge stools have irreversibly changed the digestive organ.

Hemorrhoidal infection and butt-centric gaps: A low fiber diet is critical to the prevention and treatment of these two conditions (brought about by huge, hard stools, and the stressing needed to oust them) and their various reactions.

Fractious gut disorder. A low fiber diet alleviates IBS symp-toms when huge stools "leave" the gut. No aggravation inside the entrail approaches no touchy gut. It's as straightforward as that.

Crohn's disease. Crohn's illness is IBS gone excessively far. A low fiber diet is critical to treating and preventing Crohn's sickness.

Ulcerative colitis. This shocking illness is the straw that broke the camel's back—the aggregate of the entirety mentioned above. Normally, the treatment of ulcerative coli-tis must start with a zero fiber diet to wipe out its diarrhea, clogging, and irritation causing impacts.

Diseases of the stomach related organs: A low fiber diet lessens the stomach-related system's odds of getting struck by the disease. It wipes out the significant dietary reason for stomach-related issues. Commonly, solid organs are less inclined to get influenced by ma-lignancies than undesirable organs. The terrible reality that ulcerative colitis expands the danger of colon malignancy 3,200% pro-vides us with all the confirmation we need about the fiber disease connec-tion.

A low fiber diet alone isn't an assurance of dynamic health and limitless life span. It is significant progress toward attaining these prized things. Besides profiting your digestive system, a low fiber diet does some incredible things for your endocrine system and digestion.

The metabolic focal points of a low fiber diet

While the endocrine system oversees the digestion of vitality, it's you who administers the flexibility of supplements that give the energy in any case. Genuine separation of digestion is an extraordinariness: just about 5% of diabetes casualties, for instance, experience the ill effects of a disappointment of the pancreas to deliver insulin. The other 95 percent overpower the body with endless starches that their pancreas either can't stay aware of the interest (for insulin), or their bodies sim-ply overlook the insulin, which is as of now copious.

Subsequently, genuine recuperation from metabolic issues like diabetes lies not in consuming more medications to deceive the pancreas into delivering much more insulin or burdening the liver into changing overabundance glucose into considerably more muscle versus fat, yet in balance.

The plain, basic, elemen-tary balance between how much energy you truly need and the amount you're getting from food.

Many people can't find that balance, not because they aren't will-ing, or are silly, however, because they're deceived about the function of dietary sugars and common fiber in health and nu-trition. That is the reason so some benevolent and health awareness indi-viduals favor getting their fiber from plentiful "regular" sources, trusting it's healthier while, in actuality, it's as a long way from reality as New York is from Paris.

Regular fiber—both the soluble and insoluble kind—is available just in a plant-based diet, for example, grains, nuts, seeds, vegetables, organic products, and vegetables. Likewise, it's found in nourishments handled from these plants, for example, grains, bread, pasta, and heated stock.

Most of these diets contain somewhere in the range of five to multiple times more carbohy-drates than fiber, which is sufficient to overwhelm even the most ro-bust endocrine system with overabundance vitality. Along these lines, when you cut down on the fiber-rich nourishments in your eating regimen, you're likewise removing ac-companying carbs, and bringing the vitality gracefully and request once again into balance.

Expecting you won't race to replace these avoided carbo-hydrates with refined sugar, natural product juices, and sodas, your eating routine will get low in fiber, however determinedly low in carbs also. In this way, fortunately, you'll be gathering the advantages of a low-carb diet, as well.

Meanwhile, carbs (for example, mono and disaccharides, for example, sugar) di-gest quickly and cause a short spike in glucose, complex carbs (such as polysaccharides.

For example, starches in grains) digest for quite a long time at once. From the start, while absorption is occurring, the pan-creas secretes insulin to stay aware of the consistent flexibility of glucose entering the circulatory system.

A constantly raised degree of insulin is called hyperinsulinemia. Other than incredibly uncommon pancreatic tumors and different problems, there is just one factor that can cause hyperinsulinemia: dietary car-bohydrates. The more carbs you eat, there is a chance of more insulin production to use them.

Raised insulin is a strong vasoconstrictor, limiting major and minor veins all through the body. When this hap-pens, circulatory strain, and heartbeat rates go up, oxygenated blood flexibly conveyed to the basic organs and limits goes down.

Hence, hyperinsulinemia is an essential driver of raised pulse, coronary illness, atherosclerosis, diabetes, liver disorder, kidney disappointment, nerve harm, visual deficiency, fringe vascular sickness, dementia, headache, cerebral pains, interminable weariness, attention shortfall or hyperactivity issue, hypoglycemia (low glucose), unending craving, and heftiness. Also, that is only the large ones.

Quite recently, the total of a large portion of these indications was called Syndrome X. Presently, it's designated "prediabetes" because the "X" in disorder is not, at this point, a riddle. It represents hyperinsulinemia, which is brought about by many such starches in one's eating regimen. Consider a normal "sound" breakfast:

- A Glass Of Squeezed Orange (26 G Of Carbs)
- Some Kellogg's Crispix (25 G) With Some Milk (12 G)
- One medium-sized Banana (27 G)

That is 90 g of carbs, or what could be compared to six tablespoons of sugar, which is al-most a large portion of the day by day requirement for the normal grownup. While this breakfast continues processing, the body continues discharging insulin, practically a large portion of the everyday portion. Furthermore, that is, before a few bites, soft drinks, lunch, and supper.

If you don't expend massive carbs measures, the pancreas doesn't flood your body with insulin. So when your utilization of carbs goes down, the condition of your health goes up, and you can hope to see the accompanying increases just from handling the hyperinsulinemia:

Hypoglycemia: At the point when glucose drops down under 40–50 milli-grams per deciliter of blood (mg/dl), an individual loses consciousness (for example, extreme lethargies, syncope).

It may regularly die not from the coma state itself, yet the following mishap. For example, a fall or fender bender. Hypoglycemia happens when more insulin is in the system than accessible glucose to fulfill de-mand by the focal sensory system. Its manifestations are difficult to miss: weakness, laziness, crabbiness, hunger, migraine, cognitive decline, vision aggravations, discourse disability, precariousness, dizzi-ness, shivering in the hands, or lips, widened students, fast heartbeat, low pulse, and some others. At the point when insulin levels are typical, hypoglycemia isn't probably even on a zero-carb diet, because the body can keep up a consistent degree of blood glucose from different sources of vitality, for example, dietary fats and proteins, or put away en-ergy as glycogen in the liver, fat from fat tissue, protein from muscle tissue, etc.

Raised fatty acids: A significant level of fatty acids is viewed as a more target marker of propelling coronary illness than some other factor. When starches are decreased, the degree of fatty oils sticks to this same pattern, because the liver no longer needs to change over the overabundance of blood glucose into fatty oils, which, inciden-tally, becomes muscle versus fat. Incessantly raised fatty substances in-crease blood thickness, which is another significant reason for the raised circulatory strain.

Hypertension: Your circulatory pressure will standardize because insu-lin no longer clog your veins and no longer powers your heart to supply more blood to conquer the obstruction of restricted vessels just as gooey (from triglyc-e-rides) blood.

Coronary illness: Your heart condition will improve because your heart muscles will get all the more all-around oxygenated blood. Furthermore, be-cause it won't need to siphon the blood extra difficult to conquer the neutralization of contracted veins and the grating brought about by fatty oils.

Atherosclerosis: If you experience the bad effects of atherosclerosis, it might gradu-ally switch itself since insulin no longer adds to vascu-lar dangerous infection, which harms the vessels on the in-side and prompts the gathering of vascular plaque—an essential driver of lasting narrowing of the influenced vessels.

Headache cerebral pains: The two most conspicuous dietary causes be-hind headache migraines are the narrowing of cerebral blood ves-sels by insulin and cerebral edema brought about by an abundance of dietary potassium.

Sugar rich nourishments are on the double the biggest source of dietary potassium and the triggers of insulin. A low-carb diet is the best migraine "medication." Alcohol, monosodium glutamate (MSG), normally happening and included sul-fites in wine. The corrosive amino tyramine is found in wines, cheeses, and numerous different nourishments are additional triggers for head-aches, random to insulin or sugars. When these are included in the head of such a large number of carbs, a cerebral pain can become a big headache.

The inability to concentrate: This condition is brought about by im-paired cerebral dissemination, low glucose, and general fatigue. These three elements push down the central nervous system (CNS) and interfere with ordinary everyday capacities and activities. Consideration deficiency/hyperactivity issue (ADHD) in kids.

Since both raised glucose and insulin are intense energizers of the CNS, kids react to them by substituting hyperactivity and exhaustion cases. The two states interfere with fixation and cause standards of conduct that are viewed as abnormal. Soon after influenced youngsters are set on a low-carb diet, the manifestations of ADHD slowly decrease, and in the long run, disappear. It just requires some investment for a kid's pancreas to decrease the produc-tion of insulin and adjust to another example of conduct.

Sleep deprivation. A blend of raised degrees of insulin (a vitality hormone) and raised degrees of glucose (fuel for CNS) are the essential drivers of useful (for example, reversible) restlessness. How might one rest when the body is so overstimulated with en-ergy? That is the reason you've been advised by your elders not to eat se--veral hours before sleep time.

As individuals get more established, processing and utili-zation of vitality extend from the standard 4–6 hours to 8, 10, or even 12 hours. So regardless of whether you've finished your supper by 7 p.m., it might keep processing until 3, 5, or even 7 a.m. When you finally snooze off, the rest is shallow because the degree of insulin stays high long after the glucose has gone down. Of course, the nature of the rest goes up when the measure of dietary carbs goes down. Similarly, as with ADHD, it takes some effort to tame and alter the unlimited (not subject to the eating regimen) influx of insulin.

Interminable Fatigue Syndrome: A blend of fatigue from low glucose, mental and strong unresponsiveness identified with clogged veins (deficient flexibly of blood), and general weari-ness originating from ongoing sleep deprivation are the essential ingredients of constant weakness condition.

The decrease of dietary starches takes out the reasons for low glucose, bloodvessel narrowing, and sleeps deprivation, and brings invited vitality back. If this doesn't happen, search out and dispose of other potential causes, such as celiac sickness, sickliness, lack of hydration, low thyroid capacity, interminable contaminations, immune system issues, sadness, etc. Of course, a high-carb diet contributes powerfully to every one of these conditions.

Vulnerability to colds: A raised degree of glucose in sound kids stimulates metabolic rates and raises internal heat level, which causes excessive sweat. At the point when kids sweat, they're bound to get chills from the resulting fast evapora-tion—a condition that makes them helpless to colds. Grownups may get colds for comparative reasons, then again, actually, for their situation, con-stricted veins lower internal heat level and encourage bacte-rial contaminations.

Also, raised blood glucose degrees to give extensive feed to fledging microorganisms to attack, multiply, and overcome youngsters and grownups' safe arrangement. The abundance of carbs makes you a mobile Petri dish, prepared and ready to shelter, feed, and develop any bacterial microbe that happens to be near. A decrease of dietary sugars in the eating routine essentially lessens the opportunity of bacterial contaminations.

Skin inflammation or acne: Hormonal changes in youngsters has little to do with skin break out. Adolescence happens to coincide with the presence of completely func-tional sebaceous glands all over and body. Abundance oil ex-creted by these organs obstructs them, while the microbes held up inside them causes contamination and emission. A zero-carb diet is one of the best methods for skin inflammation control because it checks oil creation by lessening the degree of fatty oils in the blood.

It doesn't invigorate bacterial development as much be-cause of a decrease in the degree of glucose.

Seborrhea: Other than "dandruff," the term seborrhea signifies "a lot of oil." A low-carb diet controls seborrhea for the equivalent rea-sons it "treats" skin break out: it wipes out overabundance fatty oils (got from glucose and aging of fiber), which are the main source of "an excess of oil." The fats from plant oils found in dressings and mayonnaise additionally add to seborrhea and skin inflammation. A low fiber diet, alongside a moderate utilization of es-sential fats from creature sources, helps control dandruff and skin break out without falling back on clinical medicines.

Fungal disease: Candida albicans, a yeastlike parasite, is com-monly present in the mouth, vagina, and intestinal area. In sound individuals, its expansion is monitored well by sym-biotic microscopic organisms and other safe cofactors.

It's accepted that a de-ficiency of nutrients B12, folate, zinc, and selenium adds to candidiasis, an irregular organism's irregular development. This development is fur-ther continued by a raised degree of glucose. Intestinal in-flammation brought about by gluten (a wheat protein), and the fermenta-tion of fiber (a source of raised causticity) are the two essential drivers of nutrient and mineral inadequacies even among individuals who take supplements or eat an "adjusted" diet. A decrease of car-bohydrates (particularly from the grain gathering) and the elimina-tion of fiber is viable protection from repeating fungal infec-tions, particularly when joined with quality enhancements.

Liver sickness: A condition known as greasy liver, which is brought about by the constant attack of sugars, is reversible in peo-ple who embrace a low-carb diet.

Its inversion incredibly benefits the individuals who have been influenced by hepatitis because a sound liver has a serious extent of protection from these viruses.

Diabetes Type II: If you have diabetes type II (noninsulin depend-ent), its side effects should slowly invert. You might have the option to get off reactions inclined medicine because glucose's normali-zation is a practically quick reaction to a low-carb diet. Try not to pass judgment on your recuperation progress just on self-testing or fasting plasma glucose tests. Take the HbA1c (glyco-sylated hemoglobin) test. Not at all, like the fasting plasma glucose test, which takes an immediate preview of the broadly fluctuating day by day levels of glucose, the HbA1c mirrors the normal concentra-tion of glucose in the blood during the first six to about two months. It presents a genuine image of diabetes, independent of outside conditions.

For example, a quick, medicine, or ongoing feast. Sit tight for two months from the day you start a low-carb diet before stepping through this exam.

Type I Diabetes: If you have type I diabetes (insulin subordinate), you ought to have the option to fundamentally lessen your portions of insulin to a lot more secure level. As a rule, you may find that you have been misdiagnosed, that your pancreas is as yet useful, and that it can oversee glucose all alone. As per some ex-perts, the pace of misdiagnosis of type I diabetes among youngsters is up to 50%. It isn't simply raised glucose that is, in the end, hurting these kids, yet additionally, the enormous portions of insulin pre-scribed to help their high-carb eats less.

Visual deficiency: Your eyes aren't as liable to surrender to diabetic reti-nopathy, a condition generally identified with diabetes, hypertension, hyperinsulinemia, and raised fatty oils, and the main source of visual impairment among grownups with either sort of diabetes, and (considerably more regularly) with undiscovered diabetes.

Infertility. A low-carb diet may support your moxie similarly just as Viagra does because the two things widen and loosen up the blood ves-sels that administer erections. Likewise, in contrast to Viagra, a low-carb diet won't cause migraines or visual impairment. On the off chance, it wasn't to shield individuals from spoiling their health and get individuals far from having intercourse, even with their true life partners.

Nerve impairment. Lowcarb slims down to shield you from nerve impairment brought about by hyperinsulinemia. Diabetes and prediabetes related nerve harm are related to lost affectability in the ex-tremities. Nerve impairment of the butt-centric waterway is an essential driver of clogging and reliance on fiber to move the bow-els. Punitive and vaginal nerve impairment influences intercourse be-cause the casualties can't hit a climax. Untimely ejacula-tion likewise results from wrong overstimulation of the apprehensive re-ceptors by raised insulin. That equivalent overstimulation, in the end, causes the receptor's demise.

Hunger control: Slippery yearning and ceaseless craving are many of the side effects of hyperinsulinemia, the two pro-voked by low glucose. This opiatelike impact of insulin is also difficult to survive. The desire to expend starches is past basic conscious control, yet determined by the body's sur-vival senses and unlimited reactions.

For anybody needing to shed pounds, or in any event, wishing not to increase any more weight, this exertion free checking of the craving is one of the most wonderful parts of a low-carb way of life.

Overweight: On the off chance that you are overweight, you may quit placing on weight and start to progressively lose muscle to fat ratio, since muscle to fat ratio is made al-most only from the sugars in your eating regimen. On the off chance that you con-sume under 200 g of sugars day by day (a normal for the medium-sized grownup), the parity is drawn from muscle versus fat (the physiology of weight reduction). If you expend more than 200 g, you get fatter, and fatter, and fatter.

Low weight: In case you're underweight, you may start putting on weight slowly. The blend of your hereditary qualities, insulin resis-tance, and hyperinsulinemia is the essential driver of weight reduction.

Hereditary qualities decide the capacity of your fat tissue to store fat. Hyperinsulinemia causes insulin obstruction or cells' inabil-ity to react to the insulin signals to begin engrossing glucose. Like this, this metabolic issue turns on lipoly-sis (a change of muscle versus fat into vitality) and gluconeogene-sis (a metabolic capacity that produces glucose from muscle tissues). The concurrent powerlessness to aggregate fat, and the utilization of muscle to fat ratio and muscle tissues for vitality, cause weight reduction and forestalls weight gain. The cycle is like the weight reduction experienced by individuals with type I diabetes, ex-cept for their situation. The raised insulin originates from the infusions.

Kidney disease: If you have a kidney disorder, you'll see an im-provement for two reasons: (1) When the degree of glucose in the blood surpasses 200 mg/dl, the hyperosmotic pressure powers the kidneys to sift through abundance sugar with pee.

(2) Hyperinsuline-mia causes expanded circulatory strain, which demolishes sensitive kid-ney tissues. The joined assault of the two powers (hyperosmo-tic weight and circulatory strain) doesn't allow the kidneys to recover and recuperate from the first harm.

Nighttime Polyuria: You'll no longer outfit in the night to pee as regularly, if by any means. Kids, whose rest is such a great amount of more profound than that of grownups, aren't as liable to have embar-rassing scenes, either. Bedwetting and evening pee oc-cur due to two elements: (1) raised degrees of glucose cause hy-perosmotic pressure and a correspondingly high pee yield; and (2) a continuous inclination is brought about by incendiary bladder dis-ease, coming about because of raised degrees of corrosiveness and glucose in the pee. The two conditions add to bacterial contamination of the blad-der and resulting irritation.

Cancer: Colon Cancer, analysts decided an immediate association between the addition of dietary car-bohydrates and malignant growth. All malignancies start with only one cell. The probability of this cell grabbing hold and developing into an all-out tumor increment considerably when the immune system is smothered by dysbacteriosis, via starch related issues, and when blood flow is hindered by hyperinsulinemia. Additionally, it's a verifiable truth that (glucose) is an essential metabolic fuel for destructive cells: the more glucose in the sys-tem, the quicker the expansion of essential malignancy and optional metastases. When the assault of carbs is switched, the green-house conditions for tumors are additionally turned around, anyway indirectly.

How much fiber do you need?

The Institute of Medicine, which gives science put together counsel concerning medication and wellbeing issues, gives the accompanying everyday fiber plans for grownups. If you aren't getting enough fiber every day, you may need to support your demand with some fiber-rich diet. Great decisions include:

- Whole grain items
- Natural products
- Vegetables
- Beans, peas, and different vegetables
- Nuts and seeds

Refined or handled diet —, for example, canned foods are grown from the ground, mash free squeezes, white bread and pasta, and grain oats — are lower in fiber. The grain refining measure eliminates the grain's external coat (wheat), which brings down its fiber content.

Improved nourishments have a portion of the B vitamin and iron included back after handling, yet not the fiber.

Fiber supplements and a refreshed diet

The entire diet, as opposed to fiber supplements, is commonly better. Fiber supplements, for example, Metamucil, Citrucel, and FiberCon — don't give the variety of strands, nutrients, minerals, and other productive supplements that diet does. Another approach to get more fiber is to eat food, for example, grain, granola bars, yogurt, and frozen yogurt, with fiber included. The additional fiber typically is named as "inulin" or "chicory root." Some individuals grumble of gassiness after eating food with included fiber.

Be that as it may, a few people may even now require a fiber supplement if dietary changes aren't adequate or have certain ailments, such as blockage, the runs, or badtempered inside condition.

Check with your PCP before taking fiber supplements.

Tips for fitting in more fiber

Need thoughts for adding more fiber to your dinners and snacks? Attempt these suggestions:

- Kickoff your day for breakfast, pick a high fiber breakfast grain — at least 5 grams of fiber a serving. Pick oats with "entire grain," "wheat," or "fiber" in the name. Or then again, include a couple of tablespoons of natural wheat grain to your chosen oat.

- Switch to whole grains. Expend in any event half of all grains as whole grains. Search for bread with whole wheat, whole wheat flour, or another whole grain as the main fixing on the name and has at any rate 2 grams of dietary fiber a serving. Switch with earthy colored rice, wild rice, grain, wheat pasta, and bulgur wheat.

- Build up cooked stock. Substitute wholegrain flour for half or the entirety of the white flour when heating. Have a go at including squashed grain oat, natural wheat, uncooked cereal to biscuits, cakes, and treats.

- Incline toward vegetables. Beans, peas, and lentils are a phenomenal source of fiber. Add kidney beans to canned soup or a green plate of mixed greens. Alternatively, make nachos with refried dark beans, heaps of new veggies, entire wheat tortilla chips, and salsa.

- Eat more products of the soil. Products of the soil are plentiful in fiber, just as nutrients and minerals. Attempt to eat at least five servings day by day.

- Make the most of snacks. New natural products, crude vegetables, low-fat popcorn, and entire grain saltines are, for the most part, great decisions. Additionally, a modest bunch of nuts or dried organic products is a solid, high fiber snack — even though they know that nuts and dried natural products are high in calories.

- High fiber nourishments are useful for your health. Be that as it may, including many fibers excessively fast can advance intestinal gas, stomach bloating, and squeezing. Increased fiber in your eating routine progressively over half a month can put a visible effect. This permits the normal microbes in your digestive system to acclimate to the change.
- Likewise, drink a lot of water. Fiber works best when it ingests water, making your stool delicate and smooth.

CHAPTER 5

A Fiber Fueled Microbiome

The Gut Microbiome Ecosystem

The happiness word for our environment is "biodiversity." We need to consider this since it influences any environment. It doesn't make a difference on the off chance that we discuss a huge environment like the woodland fires in Australia or the Amazon rainforest or on a tiny level within us at this moment. Our gut is as a lot of an environment as the amazon rainforest. Shockingly, something very similar that we see occurring to our timberlands is going on within us in the 21st century. We haven't been dealing with our gut! It is so intuitive when you consider it. With any biological system, it could be woodland or dirt; when we eradicate that environment's biodiversity, it loses its strength. The gut is likened to a dirt situation; it resembles having soil inside the body.

I am a plant-based person because the science that I was perusing driven me. I shed 50 pounds by following the diet that is Fiber Fueled. Be that as it may, I am not saying there is just a single solid method. I realize that we won't wake up one day, and the world will be 100% veggie-lover, BUT I couldn't imagine anything better than urge individuals to move somewhat more in the plant-based food.

How Do We Acquire The Microbiome?

Ideally, a child goes through the birth canal and, in that cycle, gets the vaginal vegetation. It is intriguing because the vaginal verdure in pregnancy will begin to change and move more like a mother's gut microbiome later in the term. On the off chance that you take an infant and track them out throughout the years when they are 23 years, they have a fullfledged grownup estimated gut microbiome. There are such numerous significant components that become an integral factor during that time.

For instance: Where is the kid playing? Outside in earth or inside in a hyper-clean home is no man's land for microorganisms.

What is the kid eating? Is it true that they are breastfed? It was created through 3 million years of human development to plan itself to continue new life. There are things about it that we don't comprehend. We currently realize that there are more than 200 varieties of Human Milk Oligosaccharides. They have zero dietary benefits for the youngster, yet they are intended to take care of the microbiome and bifidobacteria. You see the development of the bifidobacteria because of breastfeeding the youngster. The fact of the matter is that there is a weak period from the hour of birth until two and whether it is performing Csection, not breastfeeding, or giving antiinfection agents, the outcome is the equivalent in all cases:

1. The increased danger of weight gain
2. Increased danger of type 2 diabetes

3. Increased danger of immune system sickness

4. Increased danger of hypersensitive conditions

The immune system needs our gut microbiome to grow appropriately. On the off chance that we disturb it during that weak timeframe, those things will continue into adulthood. Presentation to these organisms is what will prepare a safe system. It needs information to prepare B cells and T cells and necessities to connect with these microorganisms. I think we see a predominance of these autoimmune dysfunctions since we have sanitized everything. There isn't as much connection with the rest of the world or the earth to prime and train the immune system. At that point, you end up with immune system dysfunctions.

I believe that the scary thing is the young girl conceived by C Section is additionally a bottle took care of.

At that point took care of prepared nourishments, and they invest all their energy inside in a hyper sterile condition. At that point, they get ear diseases, and we shoot them with antitoxins. Both C Section conceived youngsters. We didn't like it as such; however, the two have been sound.

The Importance of Plant Foods in the Gut?

The microbiome is this network of invisible organisms that are as alive as you and me. They spread us from the head of our heads to the tip of our toes; however, they are moved in our gut. Your gut is nearly the focal point of human health. All health begins there, and it fans out. It is more than stomach related health it is:

1. Your immune system
2. Your state of mind
3. How you feel,
4. Some may contend it's even your character.
5. It is your digestion. Think about the individual who eats all the correct food and can't get in

shape contrasted with the individual who eats anything they desire, and they are as yet thin. They have a decent gut microbiome.

It is our hormones and how we express our qualities

The entirety of that is moved in this one area. Also, we have redistributed it to our microbiome. You need to upgrade those organisms to play in support of yourself, and you need to consider your life extended out more than 80100 years. You can do an eating regimen for three months, and it won't kill you in 3 months. However, if you are one of the individuals who have a cardiovascular failure in their 50's, you'll always be unable to reclaim how you did that diet. That is the truth of the issue. We need to consider the eating routine that will delay our lives' life span in our 80's100's. To me, that is a mitigating diet. The way by which we achieve that is through our gut. Utilizing prebiotics.

Probiotics are the container that has living life forms.

Prebiotics is the compost for the sound calming microorganisms in our gut. There was an investigation that a prebiotic diet comprising of fructooligosaccharides: inulin, (prebiotic) consistently improved rest. At the point when you feed them, they become more grounded, different, and unload the prebiotics (dissolvable fiber, safe starch) and delivery short-chain unsaturated fats like:

1. Butyrate
2. Acetate
3. Propionate

These are the mitigating atoms. If you need to:

- Control your immune system
- Reverse defective gut
- Prevent Alzheimer's
- Prevent Parkinson's
- Improve your temperament

Get short-chain unsaturated fats. It's astonishing what they do inside the whole body from your cerebrum down to your gut. From my viewpoint, I see this association between our gut and food. When we eat fiber added nourishments (plants, seeds, nuts, entire grains), they compensate us with the cash of gut health, short-chain unsaturated fats!

It would be best if you had biodiversity to make the most advantages for your gut microbiome. At the point when we lose it, that is when infection appears. Associating biodiversity to the way that we live and eat, what is our most ideal alternative? Is a veggie-lover diet the most advantageous thing for our gut? The appropriate response in the greatest gut health study to date was no. The single most prominent indicator of a sound gut microbiome was the decent variety of plants in your eating regimen. When you have assorted variety in your eating routine, you get a decent variety in your microbiome!

A great deal of the early examinations was finished with 16s innovation, yet moving is a touch to a greater degree, a higher goal. It is currently moving to a higher goal preview of what's going on in the gut. This is called the entire genome sequencing. They utilize the Kegg information base to work out what's going on from a metabolite perspective.

It isn't the makeups of the microbiome or the makeups of your important eating regimen. What makes a difference is the metabolites. What your microbiome produces for you is what will affect. The microbiome isn't unchangeable. I like stating, and the gut is a muscle, it very well may be prepared. It might have certain qualities, and it might have certain shortcomings. If you take your shortcomings and start low and go moderate, you can prepare your gut and make that a quality. It is conceivable and versatile.

Short-chain acids are one case of postbiotics. Postbiotics meaning health advancing particles. Many people talk about the medical advantages of polyphenols. However, it's not the polyphenols in their local state. It's the polyphenols after they have been used by your microbiome that has the mending impacts.

You do not utilize 80% of the polyphenols. An exemplary model would be pomegranate. It is rich in polyphenols, yet the postbiotics that the microscopic organisms make out of these polyphenols. This evokes a ton of advantages to mitochondrial health. Different ones that are of key significance are short-chain unsaturated fats, synapses, and LPS.

LPS and Inflammation
This is additionally alluded to as bacterial endotoxin, however, more normally, aggravation. It very well may be anything from:

A poor quality, low consumes, seething irritation. The sort of thing that can cause coronary illness 40 a long time from now. Or on the other hand, it tends to be the extraordinary inverse. Somebody who doesn't know where they are is confused, and their oxygen levels are dropping. What I am portraying is an individual in septic shock. Septic shock is because of a huge flood in LPS.

Individuals don't understand that our gut, even though it is the most profound aspect of our body, is outward confronting. It is where we interface with our condition. What's more, it is the place we are generally powerless and need the most assurance. We have this divider inherent in our gut to shield us from these undesirable microbes like E.coli and Salmonella. These gram-negative microorganisms discharge the LPS.

We, as a whole, have them since they are essential for our environment. They will deliver it, yet the inquiry is, does it breakthrough to the circulatory system? The appropriate response is, what is new with the tight intersections? When we talk about broken gut, this is the thing that we are alluding to. When the tight intersections separate, you make channels between the cells that predicament and permit the arrival of this LPS into the circulation system.

How Do We Diagnose Leaky Gut?

In the clinical field, we don't recognize flawed gut; however, we do recognize dysbiosis. This portrays a state in the gut where there are three things:

Number 1: There is lost equalization in the gut. Ordinarily, this is lost assorted variety—fewer heroes all the more trouble makers.

Number 2: Increase in intestinal porousness. This is inseparable from saying a broken gut.

Number 3: Release of bacterial endotoxin.

This is all dysbiosis. Furthermore, there is not a genuine, precise test to decide this. Individuals can peer down on the declaration of "broken gut," yet dysbiosis is very similar. I would likewise alert individuals when discussing any health data to be cautious who your source is!

The microbiome research is so close that endless reviews are coming out. It isn't easy to try and stay aware of it. You have to put time into reading each day.

The microbiome space is developing. So as we move more from 16s examinations to entire genome sequencing, the goal is unquestionably more upgraded. You are going from the family level to the subspecies examination. At that point, exacerbate that with the way that we are going to rename lactobacillus. A great deal of these investigations may get outdated. This is how quick innovation is moving.

The microbiome is completely founded on innovation since we are utilizing PCs to investigate its greater part.

What Is Crushing Our Gut in the Industrial World?

Number 1: Antibiotics. They spare lives in circumstances where we need it; however, now we got into a circumstance where we presented these antimicrobial mixes generally all through our entire natural pecking order. Many antitoxins aren't originating from the specialist; they are getting through the food flexibly, generally meat. They have made sense of when you feed a creature antiinfection agents, and it gives it 15% more mass. However, what happens when you immunize the entire system with antitoxins? The meat you are spending is affecting what's going on in the microbial network in the gut.

Number 2: Rhythmicity. This is related to your circadian rhythms. The hour of the day you eat, yet also the blue light from LED screens, whether it's the vitality sparing bulbs or your PC screen around evening time, motioning to the body that it is the center of the day. It likewise smothers melatonin. (To battle this, getting daylight presentations in the day sets rhythmicity.) So the body is confused, the microbiome (which has its circadian beat!) is additionally befuddled. A clock within the mind is called the Suprachiasmatic Nucleus, which sets the entire body's circumstance. At that point, there is motioning with the genuine microbiome, too, through the quality articulation. There are contrasts in the microbiome arrangement all through the various pieces of the day. So envision the disarray in the body's clock.

CHAPTER 6

Fiber And Immune System

Gut microorganisms help your immune system, T cells create and decide the difference between danger and your body. Likewise, your gut has a significant activity of guaranteeing that no particles should go through the intestinal layer. The defective gut is where the gut's intestinal layer has been harmed, and enormous food particles or different substances can go into the body's remainder. Once inside the body, they are seen as a danger by the immune system, prompting pain, inflammation, and potential food sensitivities. Since your immune system and digestive system are interconnected and undermined, the gut can make you more feeble to get run down or become ill.

How Fiber Impacts Your Immune and Gut Health

Fiber can uphold your invulnerable health and processing by empowering ordinary solid discharge and giving the "food" for the great microorganisms in your gut to benefit from. Like every living life form, even the microbes in our bodies need fuel to endure, and the fiber in our daily diet uses fewer calories is the thing that gives that food.

This great microbe "food" is known as prebiotics, which can be found in particular sorts of fiber-rich nourishments like jackfruit, garlic, and onions. By powering the "great" gut microscopic organisms with prebiotic fiber-rich nourishments, we can advance better stomach related health, safe health, just like numerous other promising health results.

What You Can Do Daily To Support Your Immune and Gut Health

Since you know the numerous manners by which your immune and digestive systems are associated, for what reason don't we address what you can do consistently to ensure that you are doing all that you can to keep your body feeling its best.

Eat More Fiber

This should come as no surprise, yet with regards to supporting your gut and invulnerable health, ensuring that you are getting enough fiber is critical! On normal, the dietary rules suggest that you expend ~25 grams of fiber every day, so ensure you fill your plate with lots of fiber-rich nourishments like our undisputed top choice jackfruit!

Include Prebiotics

Since you see how prebiotics upholds the great microorganisms in your gut, significantly, you ensure that you are likewise adding prebiotic-rich nourishments to your eating regimen consistently.

Jackfruit is one incredible choice for getting your prebiotics in, as are garlic, onions, bananas, leeks, and asparagus.

Lessen Your Stress

Have you ever known about the gut cerebrum center? Indeed, it fundamentally is how your mind and gut speak with one another throughout the day. The gut mind hub is liable for that feeling in your stomach when you are apprehensive or focused. Keeping in mind that this wouldn't be an issue once in a while, how the vast majority encounters constant pressure today affects our general gut health. When we are focused on, we don't process our food too, which after some time, can prompt issues like the inefficiency of the gut microbes or flawed gut, which, as we probably are aware, can affect our insusceptible health and general health. So with regards to supporting your gut health, focus on certain pressure decrease — else you will truly be taking on a tough conflict.

Drink Enough Water

Any person would agree that a great many people ought to drink more water. Remaining hydrated is basic for helping the body flush undesirable poisons and keep digestion regular. So if you need to improve your gut health AND keep that cold under control at that point, drink up! With these tips close by, you will be well headed to support your invulnerable health and processing the entire year. You will be substantially more liable to kick those cool indications before they even beginning.

CHAPTER 7

Soluble Fiber Versus Insoluble Fiber

Fiber can be placed into two classifications: soluble and insoluble fiber.

Soluble fiber, such as gelatin, gum, and adhesive, disintegrates in water; insoluble fiber, for example, hemicellulose, cellulose, and lignin don't. In the body, soluble fiber breaks down and turns into a gel-like substance. Insoluble fiber generally holds its shape while in the body. Both dissolvable and insoluble fibers have significant advantages. Soluble fiber is known to assist decline with blooding (glucose) levels. It likewise assists lower with blooding cholesterol.

Insoluble fiber, then again, speeds up the section of food through the digestive system. This keeps up normality and prevents blockage.

It additionally increments fecal mass, which makes stools simpler to pass. Most plant-based nourishments contain dissolvable and insoluble fiber; however, each change's measures in various nourishments. Great sources of dissolvable fiber incorporate beans, lentils, cereal, peas, natural citrus products, blueberries, apples, and grain. Great sources of insoluble fiber incorporate nourishments with entire wheat flour, wheat grain, earthy colored rice, cauliflower, potatoes, tomatoes, and cucumbers. A few nourishments, similar to nuts and carrots, are acceptable sources of the two kinds of fiber.

CHAPTER 8

Diet With Short Chain Unsaturated Fats

Helpful microorganisms create short-chain unsaturated fats in your microbiome, and they're essential for your gut, body, and even cerebrum health. Short-chain unsaturated fats (SCFA) can be produced using all starches, however mostly from prebiotic dietary fibers that fuel the exercises of gainful microorganisms. These natural mixes have numerous significant parts in the gastrointestinal tract, and for your more extensive health.

There are a few conditions where their creation can be restricted, mainly when we don't expend enough entire plant nourishments like the Western eating routine. Subsequently, the significance of fiber can't be messed with as well.

It's found in whole plant food sources, and because it sustains the great microorganisms in your gut, it is known as a "prebiotic." You can build your own SCFA creation by expanding your admission to these dietary filaments.

Three short-chain unsaturated fats (and lactate) are discussed in this section. Microorganisms that produce them, and how they advance various parts of our microbiome, just as digestion and psychological changes

Acetic acid derivation

Acetic acid derivation helps keep your gut condition stable and supports other advantageous microbes species in your colon. Acetic acid derivation represents the most extraordinary level of SCFAs created by your gut microbes. Like this, the creation of these mixes is vital to our general health and prosperity.

It additionally features how the commensal microscopic organisms, who see your gut as home, live in concordance.

Principle makers

The acetic acid derivation is delivered generally by Bifidobacteria and Lactobacilli, however Akkermansia Muciniphila, Prevotella spp., and Ruminococcus spp. Make it as well. For instance, when you eat fiber, it goes through your GI tract to your gut, where microscopic organisms, for example, Bifidobacteria, transform it into acetic acid derivation. This SCFA would then be utilized by individuals from the Firmicutes family to make another metabolite, butyrate, which is a fundamental source of vitality for your gut cells.

Be that as it may, microbes like Akkermansia Muciniphila are not dependent on your fiber consumption explicitly.

Instead, they love a decent much on the mucins in your gut lining, which they would then be able to change into acetic acid derivation.

Capacities for the gut and body

The acetic acid derivation is a significant controller in the pH of your gut. It assists in keeping the earth stable. For instance, it helps keep the stomach acidic enough for your advantageous microorganisms to flourish and endure, hindering the deft ones from entering and staying.

For what reason are Bifidobacteria so significant for health?

The examination has demonstrated that in a newborn who is breastfed or later took care of with nourishments containing prebiotics, acetic acid derivation hinders the development of numerous typical microorganisms (the ones which can make us unwell). The impact is likewise more prominent when the gut is more acidic as well.

It likewise tries to receptors in the gut lining where it attempts to control craving and manage the quantity of fat. These receptors have significant parts in advancing the arrival of explicit gut hormones, peptide YY and GLP1, which manage our craving. Receptors catch exact synthetic substances that induce a reaction in the body. When these hormones are delivered by cells in the small digestive system, you no longer feel hungry. In this way, you are less disposed to bite and take on additional calories. Like this, the acetic acid derivation created from the breakdown of fiber can even assist secure you against pointless weight gain.

The acetic acid derivation, created by microorganisms, such as Bifidobacteria, helps sustain the butyrate delivering organisms in your gut, supporting the decent variety of your gainful organisms. Hence, this SCFA causes different species to flourish and endure, conduct called cross taking care of.

Butyrate

Butyrate is significant for the health of our digestive system and disease anticipation, including neurological conditions. This SCFA has created not precisely the others. However, research shows that it's essential for your health. It's extraordinary to fight inflammation, which is a developing issue these days since it harms the body and builds the danger of a few constant infections.

Expanding your demand for prebiotic dietary fiber is a simple method to increase butyrate creation in your gut. It may merely check gut dysbiosis (awkward nature in your microbiome) connected to numerous sicknesses, stomach issues, and even psychological health.

Fundamental makers

Individuals from the Firmicutes family are known for making this SCFA.

The fundamental makers of butyrate are anaerobic microscopic organisms like Faecalibacterium Prausnitzii, Eubacterium Rectale, and Roseburia spp. Anaerobic microbes are types that make due in regions where no oxygen is available. Thus, in people, they are regularly found along the gastrointestinal tract. It wasn't easy to develop them in Petri dishes since they can't make due in oxygen-rich conditions.

Capacities for the gut and body

Butyrate has numerous capacities in both the gut and the body. One of its vital jobs is a primary vitality hotspot for the phones coating the gut called "colonocytes." Butyrate gives up to 90% of its all-out energy necessities. These cells need this SCFA to do their significant capacities, particularly protecting the gut lining's trustworthiness. Your gut lining is excessively substantial because it goes about as a hindrance between your intestinal condition and the remainder of your body.

When the coating is working successfully, it permits helpful things like nutrients and minerals to enter the circulation system and advance toward different body pieces that need them. Simultaneously, it stops harmful microbes, poisons, and food parts from getting into your blood and making you sick.

For what reason is Akkermansia so significant for health?

The boundary is comprised of tight intersection proteins that control the opening and shutting of the layer. However, on the off chance that these intersections can't close, it can cause a broken gut phenomenon. Yet, by having a more noteworthy bounty of butyrate makers, you will have increased production of this SCFA, which implies you'll be shielded from the cracked gut. Another extraordinary thing about this result of fiber breakdown is that it has cell reinforcement and anticancer properties.

Also, it has a genuinely cool method of doing it, as well: it makes unusual cells death themselves and keeps malignancy from happening.

However, for you to encounter the advantages of butyrate, there's something you have to do: eat more fiber. An eating routine low in entire plant nourishments implies you have less security against a bad gut and different infections, including malignant growth.

Part of psychological wellness

Butyrate is a multifunctional particle since it isn't just gainful for gut health. It's extraordinary for the mind. Eating a routine high in fiber is known to have constructive outcomes for our memory, awareness, and sensory system. Butyrate works using the gut mind center, a two-way correspondence system between the two organs.

It targets many similar pathways related to cerebrum related conditions and is thought to have numerous neuroprotective impacts.

Subsequently, if you eat a high fiber diet, you can support butyrate delivering microscopic organisms' movement. This could help protect against neurodegenerative sicknesses like Alzheimer's and Parkinson's and emotional wellness issues and chemical imbalance.

Propionate

Even though it's less concentrated than different SCFAs, propionate has some particular medical advantages that show it shouldn't be thought little of. Like the various SCFAs we've referenced, propionate is another result of dietary fiber's bacterial breakdown. It has numerous medical advantages.

Principle makers

Propionate structures when starches are separated by microscopic organisms, including those from the Bacteroidetes, Firmicutes, and Lachnospiraceae phyla. Nonetheless, the principle bacterial makers in your gut are Bacteroides Eggerthii, Bacteroides Fragilis, and Veillonella Parvula. Curiously, there are two types of Lachnospiraceae, which can create either butyrate or propionate when they are benefited from various substrates like glucose or lactate.

Capacities for the gut and body

Propionate is health advancing SCFA, which has cholesterol bringing down, diminished fat stockpiling, against disease, and calming properties. It's a result of bacterial reproduction in your internal organ. As an ever-increasing number of individuals overall are determined to have stoutness, propionate is getting expanding consideration for its likely part in stifling craving.

Much the same as acetic acid derivation, propionate likewise animates the arrival of the hormone's peptide YY and GLP1, revealing to us when we feel fulfilled after food.

What's new with gut microbes and weight gain?

In one investigation, when members were managed propionate, these craving hormones' degrees diminished vitality consumption by 14% at a choice dinner. What's more, in another investigation, weight gain was reduced by very nearly a quarter in overweight grownups over a 24week time frame where the members were enhanced with propionate.

SCFAs give fuel to the body's capacities and other microorganisms as well. Propionate delivered in your gut likewise has calming impacts all through the body.

That implies it can shield you from different ailments, including atherosclerosis, a condition where fatty plaques adhere to your corridor dividers. On the off chance that these are left undetected, they can cause blockages in the veins, expanding the danger of coronary episodes and strokes.

Much like butyrate, propionate is also accepted to have a defensive function against colon malignant growth. Even though the last is more effective because it gives vitality to the colon's cells, propionate is encouraging. Studies have indicated that it is additionally ready to cause malignant cells to end it all, essentially, keeping the disease from creating. Like this, close by butyrate, it is viewed as a strong SCFA. On the off chance that you were a malignant growth cell, you likely wouldn't have any desire to interfere with it!

Lactate

Lactate isn't a short-chain unsaturated fat; however, it's created by gut microbes and has significant responsibilities to your colon's health. Like SCFAs, lactate is a microbial metabolite. As it were, a portion of the microbes dwelling in your gut produce lactate close by different SCFAs through the breakdown of carbs. It assists with advancing your gut's soundness, and the microscopic organisms that produce it can shield you from the sickness.

Principle makers

The principal makers of lactate are lactic corrosive microbes or Lactobacillus. Or maybe supportively, the sign is in the name. Lactic corrosive microbes have been utilized for quite a long time to age nourishments, a cycle that additionally safeguards them.

Today, numerous nourishments are made with Lactobacillus's assistance, and these microscopic organisms are known for their capacity to profit our health. You're most likely acquainted with the yogurts, milk, cheddar, and kefir items on the store racks. Lactobacillus itself is a significant individual from your gut microbiome because it assists with shielding you from hurt. It even transfers substances to keep microbes from setting up camp in your gut.

Capacities for the gut and body

Much like acetic acid derivation, lactate can likewise be utilized by certain bacterial species to deliver butyrate. Thus, by keeping your Lactobacillus plenitude up, it can build the creation of lactate. Consequently, you will be, in a way keeping up the trustworthiness of your gut lining and even diminish irritation by supporting your butyrate makers. It likewise has the right parts in your immune system.

For instance, it can go about as a middle person to create both star and calming cytokines. In the gut, lactate assists with decreasing aggravation.

For what reason is Lactobacillus so significant for health?

It does this by bringing the measure of harm down to the phones covering the gut, stifling the arrival of supportive of provocative substances like IL6, and limiting the indications of irritation itself. Furthermore, to think this has just been found as of late is intriguing.

Exercise is additionally known to expand the wealth of lactic corrosive microbes. These organisms join to the coating of the gut, which is why they have significant parts in intestinal resistance and rejection of entrepreneurial microbes.

Role in emotional health

Your gut and cerebrum are connected through many nerves and nerve cells that pass motions toward and fro. Henceforth, your gut microbiome can significantly impact your focal sensory system and the flagging pathways in your mind. Exploration shows that a few microorganisms answerable for delivering lactate can improve mental wellness. They likewise add to fewer indications of sorrow. Expanding your admission of fiber can have numerous positive advantages for your temperament and cerebrum health. Short-chain unsaturated fats are the actual results of the breakdown of non-absorbable sugars by gut microorganisms. They are a significant source of vitality for colon cells, and we can expand the creation of these health advancing mixes by increasing our utilization of fiber.

Acetic acid derivation, butyrate, and propionate are the principle SCFAs delivered through bacterial maturation. In any case, lactate, even though not authoritatively a sort of SCFA, is a result of the starch breakdown by lactic corrosive microbes, and it has various medical advantages. Butyrate and propionate are particularly respected for their health advancing advantages. For instance, butyrate is notable for its enemy of malignancy properties, while propionate encourages us to feel full after eating and brings down cholesterol.

The incredible thing is, it's overly simple to expand the creation of these health advancing metabolites. You simply need to pack in the fiber. The Western eating routine is generally low in plant-based nourishments, but your body is shouting out for them. Instead, the greater part of us picks comfort nourishments that have minimal dietary benefit.

Be that as it may, by guaranteeing we add dietary fiber to every feast, we will be sustaining our gut microscopic organisms, and they'll adore you for it. As a demonstration of thankfulness, their number will develop, and their creation of SCFAs will increment.

CHAPTER 9

The Biotics Game (Pre, Pro, Postbiotic)

When the microbiome is disturbed, an entire extent of skin and other health conditions can happen, extending from dry skin and skin inflammation to stomach conditions. Thus, health and prosperity organizations are increasingly hoping to focus on the microbiome when growing new items. In general, these items and enhancements will be categorized as 1 of 3 classifications: Prebiotics, Probiotics, and Postbiotics.

Prebiotics

First authored in 1995, the term 'Prebiotics' alludes to nonabsorbable food fixings that, by definition, have a medical advantage – most generally taken orally to advance the development of useful microscopic organisms in the digestive tract.

Models incorporate parts of entire grains, bananas, greens, onions, garlic, soybeans, and artichokes. By empowering the development and movement of useful microorganisms, prebiotics like this secure and sustain our skin. Taking care of our inner parts secures our exterior!

To 'feed' our valuable gut microscopic organisms, dietary and supplement prebiotics must abstain from being processed in the stomach, giving tests, and empowering advancement in the field. Notwithstanding, prebiotics are connected to the gut and can be managed legitimately to other microbial hotspots – including the skin, with effective prebiotic skincare, a rising region in contemplates.

Just a couple of prebiotic health claims have been endorsed to date, with the genuine medical advantages of prebiotics being a source of dispute. However, who knows, we may see a greater amount of them later on!

Probiotics

With the expanding notoriety of items like Kombucha and probiotic yogurts, probiotics are maybe the most notable of the three sorts. Probiotics are characterized as microorganisms brought into the body for their helpful characteristics. As such, probiotics contain live organisms that we can add to our stable organisms to help our immune systems and dispense with microbes. The current terminology was first utilized in 1950, yet it depends on logical perceptions made sometime before in 1907.

Probiotics have much a more significant number of difficulties than prebiotics. The live microorganisms achieve numerous inquiries around health and solidness – they mustn't hurt us and must endure sufficiently long to sit on the racks and in our organizers. On the head of that, as with prebiotics, barely any health claims have been approved by administrative bodies.

Notwithstanding these issues, there is an expanding number of probiotic excellence items available – many utilizing inactivated, as opposed to living, microorganisms. In any case, many of these items are founded on parts delivered by microorganisms instead of the entire life form.

Postbiotics

Postbiotics are nonreasonable bacterial items (for example, cell divider parts) or metabolites delivered by advantageous microorganisms, for example, nutrients and lactic corrosive. As it were, they originated from the maturation (breakdown) of microbes. Practically speaking, they are made from probiotics societies that specifically impact the microbiome for more beneficial results. Consequently, numerous microbial age lysates and extricates present in probiotic beauty care products can be considered postbiotics. It is felt that the announced medical advantages of mature milk items.

For example, live yogurts, are expected more to the results of maturation than live organisms enduring absorption and applying beneficial impacts.

Investigating maturation results of microscopic skin organisms, examiners have indicated that postbiotics from skin microbes have possibly unique dynamic fixings. For example, C. acnes age may stifle network gained Methicillinsafe Staphylococcus aureus (MRSA) – a notable 'superbug' known to make troublesome treat contaminations.

CHAPTER 10

Probiotics And Fermented Foods

Probiotic-rich aged nourishments demonstrate that they can change the arrangement of the gut verdure on numerous occasions, which exhibits they are enduring. Each medical advantage recorded above depends on research explicitly looking at aged nourishments.

One examination even discovered that aged milk and yogurt were equipped to expand levels of the useful Bifidobacteria and Lactobacilli microorganisms in the colon. Yogurt additionally essentially decreased degrees of the enteropathogens E. coli and Helicobacter pylori.

Matured food probiotics are likely more steady than probiotics in pills since they contain the food fundamental for probiotic endurance – prebiotics.

I have been stating that it's ideal for getting your probiotics from matured nourishments for quite a long time. Even though there should be more investigations contrasting probiotic-rich matured nourishments with probiotics in pill structure, probiotics benefits are found in aged nourishments and enhancements.

For longer than ten years, I have been working with customers and suggesting probiotic-rich matures. In the wake of getting criticism from truly a huge number of customers, the most widely recognized outcomes individuals see are:

- Less Obstruction
- Better Processed Stools
- Fewer Sugar Cravings
- Getting No Colds And Sicknesses
- More Vitality
- Less Bloating

CHAPTER 11

Diversity Of Fiber And Its Effects

The healing properties of a low fiber diet

The effect of a low fiber diet on the stomach related cycle is recogniz-able from the moderately quick decrease of practical (re-versible) reactions brought about by overabundance fiber: the vanishing of acid reflux (because there is less undigested food inside the sto--mach), the nonappearance of swelling (because there is less bacterial fermen-tation), the simple going of stools (because the stools are littler), the decrease of hemorrhoids (because there is less strain-ing), and the continuous evaporating of annoying stomach uneasiness (on account of the entirety of the abovementioned). You can't miss these signs.

The advancement doesn't end with simply alleviating symptoms: as the nature of processing improves, your body starts to ingest more basic supplements from basically a similar eating routine you devoured be-fore because fiber is no longer there to obstruct their assimila-tion. The improved accessibility of supplements quickens tissue regen-eration through the body, restores the endocrine sys-tem, and expands the yield of stomach related proteins. This, like this, ac-celerates the repair of the stomach related organs, which like this, im-proves processing, and thus quickens the healing process.

This cycle of recovery is the direct inverse of the mischief fiber causes. The mischief begins with fiber's obstruction with absorption: as assimilation turns out to be less proficient, so does the body's capacity to oppose hurt.

As the damage increments in scope, assimilation turns out to be even less proficient, and the mischief more obvious. This bit by bit decrease in health quickens with maturing. In that lies one more significant ad-vantage of the low fiber diet:

A Low fiber Diet Decelerates

Age-Related Decline might be moderate and vague on youngsters' account, and abrupt and clear in more established individuals. Yet, the as-pects of the decrease brought about by fiber stop the second you quit over-consuming it.

I underscore this highlight teach a portion of confidence in you: it doesn't make a difference how old you are, nor does it make a difference how far either issue has advanced. When you make a move, you shut down oneself committed bad, be-cause you eliminate one of its most conspicuous causes. In any event, this in itself, when complete recovery may not be achievable, merits the ef-fort.

Sicknesses aside, the effect of fiber's decrease on satiety is yet an-other significant bit of leeway of the low fiber diet. While craving makes you need to eat, an absence of satiety makes you indulge. The instruments behind satiety are predominantly physiological—you don't feel fulfilled from eating until the stomach is filled to a specific ca-pacity. That is the reason stomach decrease medical procedures are so successful for extremely chubby individuals: after the medical procedure, they need only a small amount of food to feel "stuffed."

In any case, we aren't brought into the world with colossal, hungry stomachs. They loosen up slowly as we continue filling them with a high mass eating regimen. Fiber advocates peddle this wonder as a bit of leeway: fi-ber tops you off and advances satiety, they guarantee.

In any case, that is a fiend's advantage, as each new "top off" continues extending your sto-mach a minuscule piece more, so whenever around, you need a small piece more food to fill it to satiety once more. Do this for certain years, and in the long run, you "grow" a stomach that is, to be sure, difficult to please. This is one more part of fiber dependence.

Luckily, it additionally works backward: when you quit consum-ing a high fiber diet, your stomach starts to steadily fade, and with each new supper, you'll require less and less food to feel fulfilled. This without a gastric detour (GBP) or a stomach band pressed around it—the two most mainstream surgi-cal choices to lessen the stomach's ability and "accelerate" sa-tiety.

CHAPTER 12

The Role Of Water

Being honest with your body as its weight is around 60% water, as indicated by the U.S. Topographical Survey. Your body uses water for its cells, organs, and tissues to assist temperature and keep up other real capacities. As a human body loses H2O through the following procedures breathing, perspiring, and assimilation, it's essential to rehydrate by drinking liquids and eating nourishments that contain water. The standard of water you rely upon is a variety of elements. The atmosphere you live in, how truly productive you are, and whether you're encountering a sickness or have some other medical issues all influence suggested admission.

1. Water Protects Your Spinal Cord, Muscle, Tissues, and Joints

Water accomplishes something other than extinguishing your thirst and direct your internal heat levels; it keeps the tissues in your body sodden. You are familiar with the feeling of your nose, eyes, and mouth dryness; sometimes, it gets irritating and unbearable. Keeping your body hydrated encourages it to hold ideal dampness degrees in these touchy territories, just as in the blood, bones, and cerebrum. Also, water secures the spinal rope, and it goes about as an ointment and pad for your joints.

2. Water Helps Your Body Remove Waste

Sufficient water consumption empowers your body to discharge squander through sweat, pee, and poop. Water enables your kidneys to eliminate squander from your blood and keep the veins that race to your kidneys open and channel them out, as per the National Kidney Foundation.

Water is additionally significant for forestalling obstruction, calls attention to the University of Rochester Medical Center. Nonetheless, as exploration notes, there is no proof to demonstrate that expanding your liquid admission will fix the stoppage.

3. Water Aids in Digestion

Water is significant for proper assimilation. Water assists in breaking down the food you eat, permitting its supplements to be consumed by your body. After you drink, both your little and digestive organs retain water, which moves into your circulation system and is additionally used to separate supplements. As your internal organ ingests water, stool changes from a fluid to healthy, as per the National Institute for Diabetes and Digestive and Kidney Diseases. Water is likewise essential to assist you with processing solvent fiber, per Medline Plus. With the assistance of water, this fiber goes to gel and eases back absorption.

4. Water Prevents You From Becoming Dehydrated

Your body loses liquids when you participate in vigorous exercise, sweat in high warmth, or catch a fever or agreement an ailment that causes heaving or lose bowels, as per the Centers for Disease Control and Prevention. In case you're losing liquids for any of these reasons, it's imperative to build your liquid admission so you can reestablish your body's characteristic hydration level. Your PCP may likewise prescribe that you drink more liquids to help treat other health conditions, similar to bladder diseases and urinary plot stones. In case you're pregnant or nursing, you might need to talk with your doctor about your liquid admission because your body will utilize more liquids than expected, particularly in case you're breastfeeding.

5. Water Helps Your Brain Function Optimally

Ever feel foggy-headed? Taste water. Exploration shows that lack of hydration is a drag to memory, consideration, and vitality. It is per a little report on grownup men from China distributed in June 2019 in the International Journal of Environmental Research and Public Health. It's no big surprise, considering H2O makes up 75 percent of the mind, the creators call attention. One explanation behind that foggy-headed inclination? "Satisfactory electrolyte balance is imperative to keeping your body working ideally. Low electrolytes can cause issues, including muscle shortcoming, exhaustion, and disarray.

6. Water Keeps Your Cardiovascular System Healthy

Water is a tremendous aspect of your blood. (For example, plasma — the light yellow fluid bit of your blood — is around 90% water, notes Britannica.)

If you become got dried out, your blood turns out to be more focused, which can prompt a lopsidedness of the electrolyte minerals it contains (sodium and potassium, for instance), says Susan Blum, MD, the originator of the Blum Center for Health in Rye Brook, New York. These electrolytes are fundamental for appropriate muscle and heart work. "Parchedness can likewise prompt lower blood volume, and consequently circulatory strain, so you may feel unsteady or woozy standing up.

7. Water Can Help You Eat Healthier

It might be straight, yet it's incredible. In an investigation of more than 18,300 American grownups, individuals who drank only 1 percent more water a day ate fewer calories and less immersed fat, sugar, sodium, and cholesterol, as per an examination distributed in February 2016 in the Journal of Human Nutrition and Dietetics.

Water may help top you off, mainly if you drink it before eating a feast. This thought was upheld up in a little investigation of 15 youthful, sound members distributed in October 2018 in Clinical Nutrition Research.

CHAPTER 13

Sliding Into A Plant-based Diet With Intestinal Issues

Generally, a plant-based eating regimen is an extraordinary method to improve your digestive system. It's plentiful in fiber, water, nutrients, minerals, and ailing in difficult to process nourishments, such as red meat, dairy, and eggs. However, a few people such as myself have stomach related troubles and may discover a plant-based eating regimen testing from the outset. We prefer to guarantee that there are some straightforward approaches to managing stomach related challenges, such as low stomach corrosive, heartburn, IBS, and general swelling that make things simpler.

Recollect that everybody is unique, and the ideal approach to discover the nourishments that function admirably for you is to try things out yourself. While one food may trigger issues for you, another person with stomach related battles may endure it fine. At the point when I began eating a plant-based eating routine, I plunged in with energy and educated a couple of tips for helping my assimilation simultaneously.

Those following a veggie lover eating plan can normally control their intestinal vegetation, much like their rapacious cousins. If your stomach inconveniences endure after doing the switch, check these eight hints out. They're sheltered and common, so you should lose your distress.

1. Attempt an Elimination Diet

In case you're following a vegetarian diet as of now, you may think, "Truly? Haven't I lost enough?"

However, rough getting by on a disposal diet may demonstrate that staying with it can help you distinguish your particular food triggers. While on the disposal diet, remain very much hydrated. You can confuse thirst with hunger without any problem. Finding an assortment of nourishments that don't trigger you is the purpose of such a routine, so don't stop after you distinguish a couple of food sources you can eat without inconvenience. Keep including different nourishments until you recognize one that causes an unfavorable impact.

2. Step by step Build Bean Consumption

Beans contain huge amounts of protein and filling fiber; however, they additionally contain a sugar called oligosaccharide, which the body can't process completely. This outcome in the marked gas originating from bean utilization. This isn't to state you should abandon beans — numerous veggie lovers depend on them to get a total board of amino acids.

However, bring them continuously into your eating routine. Start with half or even a fourth of the suggested serving and increment your utilization from that point. Have a go at including beans in each other or each third day from the start to continuously build your body's resistance.

3. Pick Ancient Grains

Numerous individuals experience gastrointestinal pain from gluten, a protein found in wheat. Gluten comprises of glutenin and gliadin, and the double protein makes little air rises in nourishments. Have a go at going sans grain to test if gluten is the offender behind your stomach torment. On the off chance that this facilitates your manifestations, steadily present complex starches from antiquated grains, for example, quinoa and amaranth, into your eating routine for fiber and mass. Numerous individuals, even those with the Celiac ailment, endure such grains well.

4. Stock Up on Soups

Vegetarians need a brisk get-and-go supper as much as anybody now and again; however, locally acquired prepackaged dinners regularly contain sugar, salt, and fake flavors that bother bellies. You can prepare delicious veggie-lover soups ahead of time, freeze them, and get a cup out of the cooler when you need a snappy workday to bring lunch or a simple supper. Saying "no" to locally acquired comforts instead of entire food goodness you've prepared yourself (and realize the fixing rundown to) may facilitate your desolation.

5. Back off of Crudites

Getting a bright crudites plate and stirring up some custom made French onion plunge to go with them is an extraordinary method to have a low calorie, stimulating nibble available. Be that as it may, crunchy crude veggies like broccoli and cauliflower cause gas in certain individuals.

Eating a rainbow demonstrates so useful to your health that setting aside the effort to develop a resilience bodes well. Start with little servings — think one huge floret or two medium radishes — and progressively develop your utilization to eliminate the burps.

6. Have a go at Cooking Your Veggies

Have you ever bubbled or steamed broccoli to see the water turn a greenish shade? You may filter out a portion of the supplement substance of vegetables by cooking them. However, it additionally assists break with bringing down the fiber that some who are new to veganism find irksome. Accordingly, cooking your veggies may diminish your belly inconvenience, particularly if you're new to the way of life.

Abstain from overcooking your veggies. In addition to the fact that this robs you of significant supplements, it likewise makes your vegetables limp and unpalatable — not great if you're not kidding about keeping your promise to eating savagery free.

7. Eat More Fermented Foods

Human digestion tracts contain a large group of microorganisms, huge numbers of them advantageous regarding absorption. At the point when levels of these solid microscopic organisms fall, gas, loose bowels, and stoppage happen. Be that as it may, matured nourishments recharge the body's stores of sound intestinal microbes, facilitating the hurt.

In case you're into Germanic cooking, delve into a serving of sauerkraut (less the ham or pork, obviously)!

If you incline toward Asian nourishments, check tempeh out. You can likewise drink your probiotics — kefir possesses a flavor like a veggie-lover yogurt smoothie, and fermented tea looks like a bubbly, somewhat sweet tea.

8. Take a B12 or Digestive Supplement

Your digestive organs use B12 to change over food to vitality for making red platelets, and insufficiency in this supplement can cause genuine medical issues. Severe veggie lovers are at a raised danger for B12 lack, as the supplement is found in dairy and meat items. Your PCP can recommend intravenous infusions for extreme inadequacy, or you can take an over the counter oral enhancement.

You may profit by including stomach related catalyst supplements into your eating regimen too. Many plant-based enhancements exist to reestablish a sound parity to your stomach related parcel.

Talk with your PCP on the off chance that you experience difficulty picking the correct protein supplement for your requirements.

Eating Vegan Despite Gastrointestinal Issues

There's no explanation a vegetarian diet is incongruent with the individuals who experience the ill effects of gastrointestinal misery. Indeed, numerous individuals report feeling better in the wake of following such an eating plan. By following the tips above, you can facilitate your steamed stomach while eating mercilessness free.

CHAPTER 14

Acid Reflux, GERD, And Other Gut Diseases

On the way to your stomach is a valve, which is a ring of muscle called the lower esophageal sphincter (LES). Regularly, the LES closes when food goes through it. If the LES doesn't close as far as possible or if it opens again and again, corrosive created by your stomach can climb into your throat. This can cause indications, and for example, a copying chest distress called acid reflux. If acid reflux indications happen more than two times every week, you may have an indigestion infection, otherwise called gastroesophageal reflux malady (GERD).

What are the Causes of Acid Reflux?

One normal reason for acid reflux disorder is a stomach irregularity called a hiatal hernia. This happens when the upper aspect of the stomach and LES move over the stomach, a muscle that isolates your stomach from your chest.

Regularly, the stomach helps keep corrosive in our stomach. If you have a hiatal hernia, corrosive can climb into your throat and cause indigestion sickness's side effects.

These are other normal dangerous factors for acid reflux disorder:

- Eating enormous dinners or resting directly after a feast.
- Being overweight or large
- Eating a weighty supper and lying on your back or twisting around at the midsection.
- Eating near sleep time.
- Eating certain nourishments, for example, citrus, tomato, chocolate, mint, garlic, onions, or fiery or greasy nourishments.
- Drinking certain refreshments, for example, liquor, carbonated beverages, espresso, or tea
- Smoking

What Are the prominent Symptoms of Acid Reflux Disease?

Regular manifestations of indigestion are:

Acid reflux: a copying torment or inconvenience that may move from your stomach to your mid-region or chest, or even up into your throat

Spewing forth: a sharp or severe tasting corrosive sponsorship up into your throat or mouth

Different indications of acid reflux illness include:

- Bloating
- Bleeding or dark stools or grisly retching
- Burping
- Dysphagia the impression of food being stuck in your throat
- Hiccups that don't ease up
- Queasiness
- Weight reduction for no known explanation
- Wheezing, dry hack, roughness, or constant sore throat

The remedy of acid reflux

If you sound somewhat rough and have an irritated throat, you might be preparing for a cold or an episode of this season's virus. However, if you've had these side effects for some time, they may be caused not by an infection yet by a valve—your lower esophageal sphincter. That is the muscle that controls the section between the throat and stomach, and when it doesn't close totally, the stomach corrosive and food stream once more into the throat. The clinical term for this cycle is gastroesophageal reflux; the retrogressive progression of corrosive is called indigestion.

Acid reflux can cause sore throats and dryness and may truly leave an awful intuition regarding your mouth. When indigestion produces interminable side effects, it is known as gastroesophageal reflux issues or GERD.

A widely accepted GERD indication is acid reflux—torment in the upper mid-region and chest that occasionally feels like you have a cardiovascular failure.

Three conditions—helpless space of food or acid from the throat, excessive corrosive in the stomach, and postponed stomach purging—add to indigestion. If you've been having repeated scenes of indigestion—or some other manifestations of heartburn—you may attempt the accompanying:

1. Eat sparingly and gradually

At the point when the stomach is exceptionally full, there can be more reflux into the throat. If it fits into your timetable, you might need to attempt what is now and then called "touching"— eating little suppers more as often as possible instead of three enormous dinners every day.

2. Avoid certain foods

Individuals with heartburn were once educated to kill everything except the blandest nourishments from their weight control plans. Yet, that is not true anymore. However, there are still a few nourishments that are more probable than others to trigger reflux, including mint, greasy nourishments, hot food sources, tomatoes, onions, garlic, espresso, tea, chocolate, and liquor. On the off chance that you eat any of these nourishments consistently, you may have a go at disposing of them to check whether doing so controls your reflux, and afterward have a go at including them back individually.

3. Try not to drink carbonated refreshments

They make you burp, which sends corrosive into the throat. Drink level water as opposed to shimmering water.

4. Keep awake in the wake of eating

At the point when you're standing, or in any event, sitting, gravity alone helps keeps corrosive in the stomach, where it has a place. Complete the process of eating three hours before you hit the hay. This implies no rests after lunch, and no delayed dinners or quick bites.

5. Try not to move excessively quick

Stay away from incredible exercise for a few hours in the wake of eating. An after supper walk is fine, yet a more difficult exercise, particularly if it includes twisting around, can send corrosive into your throat.

6. Rest on a slope

In a perfect world, your head ought to be 6 to 8 inches higher than your feet. You can accomplish this by utilizing "extra tall" bed risers on the legs supporting the top of your bed.

If your dozing accomplice objects to this change, have a go at utilizing a froth wedge uphold for your chest area. Try not to attempt to make a wedge by stacking pads. They won't offer the uniform help you need.

7. Get more fit if it's needed

Expanded weight spreads the solid structure that bolsters the lower esophageal sphincter, diminishing the weight that holds the sphincter shut. This prompts reflux and indigestion.

8. If you smoke, stop smoking

Nicotine may loosen up the lower esophageal sphincter.

9. Check your meds

A few—including postmenopausal estrogen, tricyclic antidepressants, and mitigating painkillers—can loosen up the sphincter, while others, especially bisphosphonates like alendronate (Fosamax), ibandronate (Boniva), or risedronate (Actonel), which are taken to build bone thickness—can disturb the throat. If these means aren't compelling or if you have extreme agony or trouble gulping, see your PCP to preclude different causes. You may likewise require a prescription to control reflux even as you seek after way of life changes.

What Is GERD?

GERD is Gastroesophageal reflux disease; it is a stomach related disturbance that influences the muscle's ring between your throat and your stomach. The lower esophageal sphincter (LES) is a ring present. If you have it, you may get indigestion or corrosive acid reflux.

Specialists believe that a few people may have it on account of a condition called hiatal hernia. As a rule, you can facilitate your GERD manifestations through an eating regimen and lifestyle changes. Yet, a few people may require a drug or medical procedure.

Causes of GERD

The expression "gastroesophageal" alludes to the stomach and throat. Reflux intends to stream back or return. Gastroesophageal reflux is the point at which what's in your stomach backs up into your throat.

In ordinary processing, your LES opens to permit food into your stomach. At that point, it closes to stop food and acidic stomach juices from streaming once again into your throat. Gastroesophageal reflux happens when the LES is frail or loosens up when it shouldn't. This lets the stomach's substance stream up into the throat.

Risk Factors for GERD

Over 60 million American grownups have acid reflux at any rate once per month, and over 15 million adults have indigestion consistently, including numerous pregnant ladies. Ongoing investigations show that GERD in babies and youngsters is more normal than specialists suspected. It can cause retching that occurs again and again. It can, likewise, cause hacking and other breathing issues.

A few specialists accept a hiatal hernia may debilitate the LES and raise your odds of gastroesophageal reflux. A hiatal hernia happens when your stomach's upper aspect climbs into the chest through a little opening in your stomach (diaphragmatic rest). The stomach is the muscle isolating the midsection from the chest. Ongoing examinations show that the opening in the stomach helps to uphold the lower end of the throat.

Numerous individuals with a hiatal hernia won't have issues with indigestion or reflux. In any case, having a hiatal hernia may permit stomach substance to reflux all the more effectively into the throat.

Hacking, retching, stressing, or unexpected physical effort can bring pressure up in your stomach and lead to a hiatal hernia. Numerous generally solid individuals over the age of 50 have a little one. Even though it's typically a state of middle age, Hiatal hernias influence individuals everything being equal.

Diet and Lifestyle Changes for GERD

There are a few changes that specialists propose you make to help reduce GERD manifestations in your way of life.

Avoid food and refreshments that triggers: Stay away from food sources that can loosen up the LES, including chocolate, peppermint, greasy nourishments, caffeine, and mixed drinks. Likewise, you should dodge nourishments and refreshments that can aggravate a harmed esophageal covering if they cause indications, such as citrus leafy foods, tomato items, and pepper.

Eat the little amount of food: Eating littler segments at supper time may help control side effects. Additionally, eating dinners in any event 2 to 3 hours before sleep time releases the corrosive in your stomach down and your stomach somewhat unfilled.

Eat gradually: Take your time at each supper.

Bite your food completely: It might help you make sure to do this on the off chance that you put your fork down after taking a chomp.

Get it again just when you've bitten and gulped that nibble.

Quit smoking: Cigarette smoking debilitates the LES. Halting smoking is imperative to decrease GERD side effects.

Lift your head: Raising the top of your bed on 6inch squares or dozing on a uniquely planned wedge lets gravity decrease the reflux of stomach substance into your throat. Try not to go through cushions to prop yourself. That alone squeezes the stomach.

Remain at a sound weight: Being overweight frequently exacerbates indications. Numerous overweight individuals discover alleviation when they get more fit.

Fiber offers high dietary benefits and is a significant factor in keeping up a sound eating regimen? In all honesty, nourishments high in dietary fiber can help counter specific ailments and sicknesses.

Other Diseases that fiber can relief

So what precisely is fiber? Dietary fiber, otherwise called roughage, incorporates all pieces of plant nourishments that your body can't process. In contrast to starches, fats, and proteins, fiber isn't processed by the body and goes practically unblemished through the digestive system.

1. Coronary illness

Coronary heart is the main enemy of the two people in America, and a high fiber diet helps bring down cholesterol. Exploration shows that ladies can diminish their danger of coronary illness by 82 percent, and men can lessen their danger by 79 percent by driving a sound way of life. Keeping up a solid, fiber-rich eating routine can improve the state of your heart. Picking an assortment of grains, particularly entire grains, just as foods grown from the ground, can decrease your opportunity of coronary illness.

2. Colon Cancer

Colon malignancy is one of the most difficult tumors for the two people. Around one of every 20 people will create colon or rectal malignancy in the course of their life. As per the American Cancer Society, an expected 26,300 men and 24,530 ladies kicked the bucket in 2013 from colon disease. Individuals with an expanded danger of malignant colon growth should make life changes to decrease their danger. Eating an assortment of organic products, vegetables, and entire grains, high in fiber and cell reinforcements, assume a part in disease avoidance.

3. Diabetes

Diabetes alludes to a gathering of sicknesses that influence how the body utilizes sugar, explicitly glucose. Glucose is vital to your health since it is an essential source of vitality for cells that make up muscles and tissue. Fiber doesn't raise blood glucose levels since it isn't separated by the body and isn't processed.

A fiber-rich eating regimen that includes a blend of solvent and insoluble filaments, similar to organic products, vegetables, entire grains, and vegetables, can improve blood glucose control and decrease cholesterol levels.

4. Constipation

Incessant clogging is inconsistent solid discharges or the trouble of passing stools that continues for a term of a little while or more. Somebody who has less than three defecations seven days is considered to have interminable obstruction. Adding fiber to your day-by-day diet expands your stool's heaviness, allowing the stool to accelerate its entry through the digestion tracts. Your primary care physician may suggest a particular number of grams of fiber for every 1,000 calories in your everyday diet.

5. Irritable Bowel Syndrome

Irritable Bowel Syndrome (IBS) is one of the most widely recognized issues of the stomach related lot and influences between 1020 percent of Americans. There is no known solution for IBS; however, soothing your side effects starts adjusting the nourishments you eat. With the endorsement of your PCP, females should join 25 grams of fiber every day into their eating regimen, and men ought to incorporate 38 grams day by day.

6. Hemorrhoids

Hemorrhoids are aroused veins in your butt or lower rectum that can be agonizing, bothersome, and now and then drain. The best strategy to prevent hemorrhoids is to keep your stool smooth. This can be practiced by eating a high fiber diet with more organic products, vegetables, and entire grains and will assist with mellowing stool and increment its mass.

Strands that relax the stool will help forestall the strain that makes hemorrhoids or intensify existing hemorrhoids.

7. Fecal Incontinence

Fecal incontinence, also called gut control issue, is the unintentional going of strong or fluid stool or bodily fluid from the rectum. Around one out of 12 individuals in America experience the ill effects of fecal incontinence. Even though anybody can experience an inside control issue's ill effects, it's generally basic among grownups. Eating the perfect measure of fiber can help with an obstruction or lose bowels related to fecal incontinence. Another regular method to treat fecal incontinence is through the utilization of fiber supplements. These enhancements can be found in drug stores or health areas of retail foundations.

8. Duodenal Ulcer

Ulcers are open wounds that happen within the covering of the throat, stomach, and the upper bit of the small digestive tract. Duodenal ulcers are situated within the upper aspect of the small digestive system. Nutrient and fiber-rich organic products, vegetables, and entire grains help the body recuperate the ulcer.

9. Dumping Syndrome

The dumping disorder happens when food, fundamentally sugar, moves excessively fast from the stomach to the small digestive tract. Manifestations of unloading disorder incorporate sickness, stomach issues, and loose bowels. They are destined to happen in people who have had a medical procedure to eliminate all or part of their stomach or have gone through a gastric detour medical procedure.

Eating five to six little, fiber-rich dinners daily, explicitly centered around grains, and disposing of sugars, such as table sugar, sweets, pop, and squeeze, will help avoid or treat unloading disorder.

10. Diverticular Disease

Diverticula are little, protruding pockets that structure the covering of the digestive system and are regularly found in the colon. Even though diverticula only here and there causes issues, they can get contaminated or excited and lead to extreme stomach torment, sickness, stoppage, or loose bowels. By devouring four to six tablespoons of coarse wheat grain a day, you can decrease material and assist it with going through the colon all the more rapidly to lessen the weight on your stomach related tract.

11. Weight Gain

Keeping up an eating routine high in fiber helps in accomplishing a sound weight.

Nourishments that are high in fiber will, in general, require additionally biting, which gives your body time to enroll that you're not, at this point, hungry. By giving your body time to enroll, you're less inclined to gorge. A high fiber feast will generally feel bigger and permit you to remain full for a more extended timeframe while devouring fewer calories.

CHAPTER 15

Fiber Fueled Everyday Meals And Recipes

1. Nectar mustard salmon with shaved brussels sprout serving of mixed greens

Fiber per serving: 5 grams

This formula is a very fun approach to switch up your pressed serving of mixed greens schedule. The brussels sprouts are high fiber vegetables and filling options in contrast to lettuce, while the cooked salmon should be served room temp, so it's ideal for grinding away.

2. 5minute lentil tomato serving of mixed greens

Fiber per serving: 9 grams

Don't you disdain suppers that take more time to plan than they do to eat? This isn't one of those. It takes 5 minutes to toss canned lentils, full cherry tomatoes, and chives in a bowl.

Keep it straightforward with simply salt and vinegar, or take an additional 30 seconds to toss in some slashed basil and garlic for significantly more flavor.

3. Singed kale and farro plate of mixed greens with salmon

Fiber per serving: 9 grams

With more fiber per serving than earthy colored rice, farro is a must-have food. This formula requires you to drench it short term before cooking, yet it's so justified, despite all the trouble. Add it on a bed of kale, top with salmon for protein, and sprinkle with sesame seeds for a lunch that tosses the "serving of mixed greens = bunny food" generalization out the window.

4. Spiced raisin and pine nut plate of mixed greens

Fiber per serving: 17 grams

This without lettuce serving of mixed greens takes the less common direction in a few different ways: from the not regular grain base to the astounding blend of curry powder, cinnamon, and turmeric to light up everything up.

In your hurry to get out the entryway, don't hold back on the flavors — they're too simple to discover, and they have a significant effect.

5. Sound chicken chickpea cleaved plate of mixed greens

Fiber per serving: 9 grams

It's tied in with energizing surfaces and flavors in this formula. Jazz up your standard chicken plate of mixed greens by tossing in certain chickpeas for additional protein, common pleasantness from corn, and a delicious chomp from the goat cheddar.

6. Marinated tempeh plate of mixed greens

Fiber per serving: 17 grams

Between the tempeh, yam, and veggies, there's sufficient fiber here for about a portion of the everyday proposal! Not decrepit for only one feast. However, noticing everything, it's actually about the smooth tahini marinade. Let your tempeh absorb it as far as might be feasible before barbecuing to get the greatest flavor.

7. Zucchini noodle Caprese plate of mixed greens

Fiber per serving of 10 grams

Chickpeas give an extra oomph to the mozzarella and tomato combo to make it a fiber-rich supper with some additional protein. What's more, with the zoodles at its base, it's fundamentally similar to eating a major bowl of pasta.

High fiber suppers with sandwiches and wraps

8. Dark bean avocado fish serving of mixed greens sandwiches

Fiber per serving: 6 grams

Neglected to pack lunch the prior night, however, truly don't have any desire to fall back on takeout? Here's something that you can arrange 5 minutes before leaving for work without holding back on nourishment or taste. Pack your bread or saltines independently for simple gathering in the workplace kitchen.

9. Turkey tortilla wrap with avocado cream

Fiber per serving: 11 grams

These wraps are made more beneficial by the trade of an avocado Greek yogurt spread rather than standard mayo. Also, the straightforward filling of tomatoes, lettuce, and turkey may return you to class days. Ok, such easier occasions.

10. Simmered red pepper, carrot, and hummus sandwich

Fiber per serving: 8 grams

In any event, something basic like changing from entire wheat cut bread to an entire wheat roll can make your common sandwich significantly additionally energizing. Slather with a sriracha spiced hummus, heap on your preferred veggies, and delve in.

11. Chickpea serving of mixed greens wraps

Fiber per serving: 11 grams

For a lighter carb feast in sandwich-like bundling, utilizing collard greens or lettuce leaves instead of bread or wraps is an incredible choice. Here, they're the envelopes for a chickpea blend that is stuffed with fiber, so you'll be full even without the grains.

12. Barbecued vegetable wrap with hummus

Fiber per serving: 16 grams

The barbecued veggie wrap is an absolute noon staple, yet numerous eatery renditions accompany much more oil and way bigger tortillas than expected. This one uses only a dash of olive oil, hummus for additional flavor, and entire wheat tortillas for a lunch that goes simpler on the fat and carbs yet at the same time figures out how to pack in loads of fiber in each serving.

13. Mediterranean barbecued chicken wrap

Fiber per serving: 7 grams

Clear, straightforward, and fulfilling: This Mediterranean formula is the ideal straightforward non-weekend day lunch, considering every contingency in one flawless bundle. While this blogger calls for cooked garlic hummus, don't hesitate to utilize your preferred assortment.

14. Green goddess sandwiches

Fiber per serving: 25 grams

We can't think about a superior name for this formula — after each of them, four of its seven fundamental fixings are green. This is one life-changing vegan sandwich with avocado, cucumbers, and fledglings tucked between thick cuts of multigrain bread.

15. Turkey, apple, and brie sandwich with apple juice mayo

Fiber per serving: 5 grams

Fresh apples, delicate brie, cut meat, and dry French bread — this is practically a cheddar plate in a sandwich structure. Pack in a decent, modest bunch of arugula for some additional fiber, and you have yourself a lunch that you'll be enticed to delve into the path before early afternoon.

High fiber plans for entrées

16. Dark beans and cauliflower rice

Fiber per serving: 15 grams

Cause one head of cauliflower to go far by beating it into a base for this without grain take on beans and rice. With a touch of sautéing, some Mexican flavors, and slashed veggies, it'll be difficult to differentiate among this and the café adaptation.

17. The best avocado pasta

Fiber per serving: 11 grams

Warmth up this pasta in the workplace microwave if you'd like; however, have confidence it's delectable cold as well. The velvety avocado sauce is rich. However, on account of heaps of fiery lemon squeeze, the dinner doesn't feel excessively substantial.

Ace tip: Make it vegetarian by excluding the Parmesan.

18. Greek quinoa bowls

Fiber per serving: 9 grams

Trade out lettuce for protein stuffed quinoa in this simple, ideal for hauling in Tupperware dish. Prepared in under 15 minutes and far better tasting once it's had the opportunity to sit, this is the ideal dinner to make ahead of time.

19. Prepared yam tacos

Fiber per serving: 11 grams

Doing without the fresh shell out and out, the yams in this formula are a higher fiber vehicle for the spiced dark bean blend. These unusual tacos do risk falling over a piece in your lunchbox; however, what's a little meddle with a supper that preferences this great and sets aside scarcely any effort to make? Bring a fork, and you'll be a great idea to go.

20. 5fixing yam dark bean stew

Fiber per serving: 9 grams

Make a huge clump of this bean stew throughout the end of the week to make your lunch an easy decision consistently. The locally acquired salsa is an alternate sound route that does the majority of the work, while storeroom flavors,

21. Entire wheat pasta with new tomatoes and spices

Fiber per serving: 8 grams

Try not to excuse pasta as only a dinnertime dish. With entire wheat pasta and new tomatoes in an olive oil dressing (rather than a weighty sauce), this is sufficiently light to appreciate for lunch without sending you into a carb actuated rest a while later.

22. Solid handcrafted moment noodles

Fiber per serving: 5 grams

Jettison the earthy colored paper sack at home for an artisan container that carries out twofold responsibility as your lunchbox and your noodle bowl in this too enjoyable to eat, more advantageous interpretation of moment ramen.

CHAPTER 16

7 Days Of Fiber Diet For Weight Loss

7Day High fiber Meal Plan for 1,200 Calories

The best is to help you get more fit, improve gut wellbeing, help your heart, lower diabetes hazard, and help you crap better.

Fiber is a sustenance demigod with some quite astounding medical advantages. Examination credits eating more fiber with weight reduction, more advantageous gut microorganisms, greater normality in your gut (otherwise known as better craps), a solid heart, and diminished diabetes danger. Anyway, if fiber can do all that, why are 95% of Americans still not getting enough? Overall, Americans just eat 16 grams of fiber daily—a long way from the 28 grams suggested in the 2020 Dietary Guidelines for Americans.

In this 7day high fiber dinner plan, your suppers and snacks for the week are gotten ready for you to make it simple and flavorful to get your fill of fiber consistently. The suppers and snacks in this arrangement incorporate many natural products, vegetables, entire grains, vegetables, nuts, and seeds; that, however, the nourishments in every class are known to have the most noteworthy fiber content—think chickpeas pear, cereal, dark beans, and chia seeds. Regardless of whether you follow this supper plan precisely or simply take a couple of thoughts to a great extent, you'll have a lot simpler time getting the fiber you have to feel much improved and remain sound.

In case you're not used to eating high fiber nourishments, bring them into your eating routine gradually and drink additional water for the day. Eating an excess of fiber excessively fast can prompt stomach squeezing.

We set this arrangement at 1,200 calories every day with changes to knock it up to 1,500 or 2,000 calories, contingent upon your calorie needs.

Step by step directions to MealPrep Your 7 days of Meals:

Day 1

Breakfast (343 calories with 12 grams of fiber)

1 serving Green Smoothie

Morning Snack (35 calories with 1 gram of fiber)

One clementine

Lunch (314 calories with 11 grams of fiber)

1 serving White Bean and Avocado Toast

1 little pear

Evening Snack (105 calories, with 2 grams of fiber)

8 dried pecan parts

Dinner (415 calories with 7 grams of fiber)

1 serving Roasted Chicken and Winter Squash over Mixed Greens

Totals: 1,211 calories, 52 grams of protein, 162 grams of sugar, 38 grams of fiber, 50 grams of fat, 1,226 mg sodium

To Make this diet of 1,500 Calories: Add 1/3 cup dry simmered unsalted almonds to morning snacks.

To Make this diet of 2,000 Calories: Include all changes for the 1,500 calorie day, also, to increase to 2 servings White Bean and Avocado Toast at lunch, addition to 1/3 cup pecan parts at evening snack, and include 1/2 an avocado to dinner.

Day 2

Breakfast (233 calories with 10 grams of fiber)

1 serving Apple Cinnamon Chia Pudding

Morning Snack (176 calories with 3 grams of fiber)

1 serving Baked Banana Nut Oatmeal Cups

Lunch (337 calories with 13 grams of fiber)

1 serving Brussels Sprouts Salad with Crunchy Chickpeas

Evening snack (77 calories on the whole)

One little apple

Dinner (401 calories with 13 grams of fiber)

1 serving Hearty Chickpea and Spinach Stew

Totals: 1,224 calories, 147 grams of starch, 155 grams of protein, 43 grams of fiber, 53 grams of fat, 1,266 mg sodium

To Make this diet of 1,500 Calories: Add one little pear to lunch and 2 Tbsp. Normal nutty spread to evening snacks

To Make this diet of 2,000 Calories: Include all adjustments for the 1,500 calorie day and increment to 2 servings Baked Banana Nut Oatmeal Cups at morning snack, include 1/2 cup low fat plain Greek yogurt for evening snacks, and include 1 serving Guacamole Chopped Salad to dinner.

Day 3

Breakfast (233 calories with 10 grams of fiber)

1 serving Apple Cinnamon Chia Pudding

Morning snack (35 calories, with 1 gram of fiber)

1 clementine

Lunch (337 calories with 13 grams of fiber)

1 serving Brussels Sprouts Salad with Crunchy Chickpeas

Evening snacks (154 calories, with 3 grams of fiber)

20 dry simmered, unsalted almonds

Dinner (464 calories, with 13 grams of fiber)

1 serving Chicken Fajita Bowls

1/4 cup guacamole, for example, Jason Mraz's Guacamole

Totals: 1,223 calories, 103 grams of starches, 67 grams of protein, 40 grams of fiber, 68 grams of fat, 1,115 mg sodium

To Make this diet of 1,500 Calories: Add 1/3 cup dry simmered unsalted almonds to morning snack.

To Make this diet of 2,000 Calories: Include all adjustments for the 1,500 calorie day and include 1 cup low-fat plain Greek yogurt for breakfast and include two servings Baked Banana Nut Oatmeal Cups for evening snacks.

Day 4

Breakfast (259 calories with 3 grams of fiber)

1 serving Baked Banana Nut Oatmeal Cups

1/2 cup lowfat12 plain Greek yogurt

Morning snack(131 calories with 7 grams of fiber)

One enormous pear

Lunch (337 calories, with 13 grams of fiber)

1 serving Brussels Sprouts Salad with Crunchy Chickpeas

Evening snacks (35 calories with 1 gram of fiber)

One clementine

Dinner (449 calories with 8 grams of fiber)

1 serving Long Life Noodles with Beef and Chinese Broccoli

Totals: 1,210 calories, 156 grams of starch, 58 grams of protein, 32 grams of fiber, 50 grams of fiber, 1,253 mg sodium

To Make this diet of 1,500 Calories: Add 1/3 cup dry simmered unsalted almonds to evening snacks.

To Make this diet of 2,000 Calories: Include all adjustments for the 1,500 calorie day and include one entire wheat English biscuit with 1/2 Tbsp. Common nutty spread and one little apple to breakfast and add 15 dried pecan parts to the morning snack.

Day 5

Breakfast (259 calories, with 3 grams of fiber)

1 serving Baked Banana Nut Oatmeal Cups

1/2 cup low fat plain Greek yogurt

Morning snack (77 calories with one gram of fiber)

Ten dry simmered, unsalted almonds

Lunch (337 calories, with 13 grams of fiber)

1 serving Brussels Sprouts Salad with Crunchy Chickpeas

Evening snacks (77 calories, with 4 grams of fiber)

One little apple

Dinner (465 calories, with 10 grams of fiber)

1 serving Slow Cooker Turkey Chili with Butternut Squash

2 cups blended greens

1/4 of an avocado, cut

One serving Maple Balsamic Vinaigrette with Shallots

Top blended greens in with cut avocado and vinaigrette

Totals: 1,215 calories, 57 grams of protein, 129 grams of starch, 39 grams of fiber, 59 grams of fat, 1,489 mg sodium

To Make this diet of 1,500 Calories: Add one medium apple to lunch and include 2 Tbsp. Regular nutty spread to evening snacks.

To Make this diet of 2,000 Calories: Include all changes for the 1,500 calorie day, in addition to increment to 2 servings Banana Nut Oatmeal Cups and 1/4 cups yogurt at breakfast and increment to 1/3 cup dry cooked unsalted almonds for a morning snack.

Supper Prep Tip: save two servings Slow Cooker Turkey Chili with Butternut Squash to have for lunch on Days 6 and 7.

Day 6

Breakfast (343 calories with 12 grams of fiber)

1 serving Green Smoothie

Morning snack (16 calories, with one gram of fiber)

1 cup cut cucumber

Spot of salt and pepper

Lunch (311 calories, with 14 grams of fiber)

1 serving Slow Cooker Turkey Chili with Butternut Squash

One clementine

Evening snacks (37 calories, with 2 grams of fiber)

One medium ringer pepper, cut

Dinner (505 calories, with 11 grams of fiber)

1 serving Butternut Squash Alfredo with Chicken and Spinach

Totals: 1,212 calories, 71 grams of protein, 148 grams of starch, 40 grams of fiber, 42 grams of fat, 1,718 mg sodium

To Make this diet of 1,500 Calories: Add one entire wheat English biscuit with 1/2 Tbsp. Regular nutty spread to breakfast.

To Make this diet of 2,000 Calories: Include all changes for the 1,500 calorie day, in addition to including 1/4 hummus and 1/3 cup dry cooked unsalted almonds for a morning snack and include 1/4 cup guacamole for evening snacks.

Feast Prep Tip: marinated the pork for Italian Roasted Pork Tenderloin with Vegetables and Quinoa, so it's prepared for supper tomorrow.

Day 7

Breakfast (259 calories with 3 grams of fiber)

1 serving Baked Banana Nut Oatmeal Cups

1/2 cup low fat plain Greek yogurt

Morning snack (37 calories with 2 grams of fiber)

One clementine

Lunch (311 calories with 14 grams of fiber)

1 serving Slow Cooker Turkey Chili with Butternut Squash

One clementine

Evening snacks (101 calories with 6 grams of fiber)

1 medium pear

Dinner (490 calories with 8 grams of fiber)

1 serving Italian Roasted Pork Tenderloin with Vegetables and Quinoa

Totals: 1,198 calories, 72 grams of protein, 153 grams of starch, 33 grams of fiber, 37 grams of fiber, 1,600 mg sodium

To Make this diet of 1,500 Calories: Add 1/3 cup dry simmered unsalted almonds to evening snacks.

To Make this diet of 2,000 Calories: Include all adjustments for the 1,500 calorie day and increment to 2 servings, Baked Banana Nut Oatmeal Cups, and increase to 1 cup yogurt at breakfast and include one entire wheat English biscuit with 1/2 Tbsp. Characteristic nutty spread to morning snack.

CONCLUSION

Fiber is a significant supplement that neglected fiber alludes to sugars that can't be processed by your gut. It is delegated either solvent or insoluble, relying upon whether it disintegrates in water. Insoluble fibers generally work as building operators, adding substance to your stool. Conversely, particular kinds of dissolvable fiber can altogether influence health and digestion — just like your weight.

An expected 100 trillion microscopic organisms live in your gut, essentially in the digestive organ. Alongside different organisms found in your digestive system, these microorganisms are regularly called the gut greenery or gut microbiome. Various types of microscopic organisms assume significant parts in different parts of health, including weight the board, glucose control, invulnerability, and even cerebrum work.

Much the same as different living beings, microscopic organisms need to eat well to remain sound.

This is the place fiber — dissolvable, generally — steps in. Dissolvable fiber goes through your digestive system generally unaltered, inevitably arriving at your neighborly gut microbes that digest it and transform it into usable vitality. The fiber that benefits your gut microbes is known as prebiotic fiber or fermentable fiber. It is viewed as exceptionally helpful for health and body weight. Gut microscopic organisms are eminent for their impact on ceaseless aggravation. They produce supplements for your body, including short-chain unsaturated fats that feed the cells in your colon.

This prompts decreased gut irritation and upgrades in related provocative issues.

Just to explain, intense (present moment) aggravation is valuable since it enables your body to battle unfamiliar trespassers and fix harmed cells. Be that as it may, constant (long haul) irritation is a significant issue since it might start to battle your body's tissues. Constant, low-level aggravation assumes a significant part in pretty much every ceaseless Western sickness, including coronary illness, Alzheimer's, and metabolic condition. There is additionally mounting proof that aggravation is related to weight increase and heftiness.

A few observational examinations exhibit that a high fiber admission is connected to bring down degrees of incendiary markers in the circulatory system. You should be in a calorie deficiency to get thinner. That is, more calories (vitality) should leave your body than entering it. Checking calories helps numerous individuals — yet it's redundant if you pick the correct nourishments. Anything that diminishes your craving can diminish your calorie admission.

With less hunger, you may get in shape without contemplating it. Fiber is regularly accepted to smother your craving. In any case, proof recommends that solitary a particular kind of fiber has this impact.

An ongoing audit of 44 examinations indicated that while 39% of fiber medicines expanded completion, just 22% decreased food admission. The gooier the fiber, the better it is at decreasing craving and food consumption. Set forth plainly, the consistency of a substance alludes to its thickness and tenacity. For instance, nectar is considerably thicker than water. Gooey, dissolvable filaments, for example, gelatins, beta-glucans, psyllium, glucomannan, and guar gum all thicken in water, framing a gel-like substance that sits in your gut. This gel eases back the purging of your stomach, expanding assimilation and ingestion times. The final product is a delayed inclination of totality and an altogether decreased hunger.

Some proof shows that the weight reduction impacts of fiber explicitly target tummy fat, which is the destructive fat in your stomach hole that is emphatically connected with metabolic sickness Fiber supplements are normally made by disengaging the fiber from plants. While these detached filaments may have some medical advantages, the proof for weight control is blended and unconvincing. An enormous survey study found that psyllium and guar gum — both dissolvable, gooey filaments — are insufficient as weight reduction supplements.

One striking special case is glucomannan, a fiber extricated from the konjac root. This unfathomably thick dietary fiber causes unobtrusive weight reduction when utilized as an enhancement. Nonetheless, enhancing with detached supplements once in a while has a lot of effects all alone.

For the best effect, you should consolidate fiber supplements with other solid weight reduction techniques. Although glucomannan and other dissolvable fiber supplements are a decent choice, it's ideal to zero in your eating routine on entire plant nourishments.

Thick strands happen solely in plant nourishments. Rich sources incorporate beans and vegetables, flax seeds, asparagus, Brussels fledglings, and oats. If you are swapping your current diet to a high fiber diet, make sure to do it bit by bit to give your body time to modify. Stomach uneasiness bloating, and even looseness of the bowels are basic symptoms on the off chance that you increase your fiber consumption excessively fast.

CPSIA information can be obtained
at www.ICGtesting.com
Printed in the USA
FSHW021253120521
81399FS